A Global Health Education Consortium Textbook

GLOBAL HEALTH TRAINING IN GRADUATE MEDICAL EDUCATION:

A Guidebook
2nd Edition

Edited by

Jack Chase, MD
Clinical Instructor
Department of Family and Community Medicine
University of California San Francisco
Hospitalist, East Bay Physicians Medical Group
San Francisco, California

Jessica Evert, MD
Clinical Instructor
Department of Family and Community Medicine
University of California, San Francisco
Medical Director, Child Family Health International
San Francisco, California

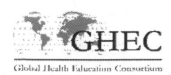

Global Health Education Consortium

iUniverse, Inc.
Bloomington

This book is supported by the Global Health Education Consortium, a non-profit organization of allied health professionals and educators dedicated to global health education in health professions schools and graduate medical education residency programs. A PDF version of this textbook is available at www.globalhealtheducation.org under Resources.

Suggested Citation: Chase, JA & Evert, J. (Eds.) Global Health Training in Graduate Medical Education: A Guidebook, 2nd Edition. San Francisco: Global Health Education Consortium, 2011. p. cm. Printed by iUniverse Publishing. ISBN 9781462007790. E-book ISBN 9781462007806.

Front cover photos (from top to bottom):
Mariel Bryden, medical student at the University of Iowa Carver College of Medicine, and community health volunteer Masakuru Keita lay a permethrin-treated bed net out to dry in Nana Kenieba, Mali. This bed net distribution project is sponsored by the NGO Medicine for Mali. (Photo credit: Benjamin Bryden.)

A row of boarded homes and storefronts in East Baltimore, Maryland – a community served by the Johns Hopkins Urban Health Residency program. (Photo credit: Rosalyn Stewart.)

Irene Pulido, Western University of Health Sciences College of Optometry second year student, performing confrontation visual field test on a patient in Bezin, Haiti. (Photo credit: Connie Tsai.)

Back cover photo:
A woman and her child in Northern Ghana pose following an interview in a qualitative research project about contraceptive use, sponsored by the Bixby Center for Population, Health and Sustainability at UC Berkeley. (Photo credit: Sirina Keesara.)

Dedication image:
Rod of Aesculapius image from Wikimedia commons, commons.wikipedia.org

Set in Times New Roman.

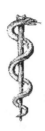

With this book, we share our hope that all people may have access to health care; that wellness becomes the standard, and disease, the exception.

Global Health Training in Graduate Medical Education
A Guidebook, 2nd Edition

iUniverse books may be ordered through booksellers or by contacting:

iUniverse
1663 Liberty Drive
Bloomington, IN 47403
www.iuniverse.com
1-800-Authors (1-800-288-4677)

ISBN: 978-1-4620-1420-0 (sc)
ISBN: 978-1-4620-0780-6 (e)

Library of Congress Control Number: 2011909738

Printed in the United States of America

iUniverse rev. date: 06/07/2011

Contents

Authors and Contributors

Kelly Anderson, MD
Resident Physician, Department
   of Family Medicine
St. Michael's Hospital
University of Toronto
Toronto, Ontario

Melanie Anspacher, MD
Assistant Professor of Pediatrics
George Washington University
School of Medicine and Health
   Sciences
Pediatric Hospitalist, Children's
   National Medical Center
Washington D.C.

David Barnard, PhD
Professor of Medicine
Director of Palliative Care
   Education
University of Pittsburgh

Tom Bodenheimer, MD MPH,
FACP
Professor, Department of Family
   and Community Medicine
Co-Director, Center for
   Excellence in Primary Care
University of California San
   Francisco

Thuy Bui, MD
Assistant Professor of Medicine
Department of Internal Medicine
Medical Director, Program for
   Healthcare of Underserved
   Populations
University of Pittsburgh
Pittsburgh, Pennsylvania

Kevin Chan, MD, MPH
Assistant Professor
Department of Pediatrics
The Hospital for Sick Children
Fellow, Munk Centre for
   International Studies
University of Toronto
Toronto, Ontario

Jack Chase, MD
Clinical Instructor
Department of Family and
   Community Medicine
University of California San
   Francisco
Hospitalist, East Bay Physicians
   Medical Group
San Francisco, California

S. M. Dabak, MBBS
Child Family Health
   International
Pune, India

S. S. Dabak, MBBS
Child Family Health
   International
Pune, India

Lisa L. Dillabaugh, MD
Fellow, Fogarty International
   Clinical Research
FACES Assistant Coordinator
Nyanza, Kenya

Paul K. Drain, MD, MPH
Fellow, Infectious Diseases
Massachusetts General Hospital
The Brigham and Women's
   Hospital
Harvard Medical School
Boston, Massachusetts

Andrew Dykens MD, MPH
Assistant Professor of Clinical
  Family Medicine
Department of Family Medicine
Director, Global Community
  Health Track
University of Illinois College of
  Medicine
Chicago, Illinois

Jessica Evert, MD
Clinical Instructor
Department of Family and
  Community Medicine
University of California San
  Francisco
Medical Director, Child Family
  Health International
San Francisco, California

Sophie Gladding, PhD
Learning Abroad Center
University of Minnesota
Minneapolis, Minnesota

Kevin Grumbach, MD
Chair, Department of Family and
  Community Medicine
University of California San
  Francisco
Chief of Family and Community
  Medicine, San Francisco
General Hospital
Director, UCSF Center for
  California Health Workforce
  Studies
San Francisco, California

Thomas Hall, MD, DrPH
Lecturer, Department of
  Epidemiology and Biostatistics
University of California at San
  Francisco
Executive Director, Global
  Health Education Consortium
San Francisco, California

Julie Herlihy, MD MPH
Boston Combined Residency in
  Pediatrics
Boston Medical Center
Children's Hospital Boston
Boston, Massachusetts

Cindy Howard, M.D., MPHTM
Associate Director, Center for
  Global Pediatrics
University of Minnesota
Minneapolis, Minnesota

Chi-Cheng Huang, MD
Assistant Professor of Internal
  Medicine
Tufts University School of
  Medicine
Adjunct Assistant Professor of
  Pediatrics
Boston University School of
  Medicine
Chairman of the Department of
  Hospital Medicine, Lahey
  Clinic
Boston, Massachusetts

Laura Janneck, MD, MPH
Resident Physician
Harvard Affiliated Emergency
  Medicine Residency Program
Brigham and Women's
  Hospital
Massachusetts General Hospital
Boston, Massachusetts

Evaleen Jones MD
Associate Professor
Stanford University School of
  Medicine
President, Child and Family
  Health International
Palo Alto, California

L. Masae Kawamura, MD
Tuberculosis Controller and
  Medical Director
Tuberculosis Control Division
San Francisco Department of
  Public Health
Co-Principle Investigator
Francis J. Curry National
  Tuberculosis Center
San Francisco, California

Daniel Philip Oluoch Kwaro,
  MBChB
Degree Candidate, MPH
University of California at
  Berkeley
Program Systems Coordinator,
  FACES

Hannah H. Leslie, MPH
Program Analyst
Department of Global Health
  Sciences
University of California San
  Francisco
San Francisco, California

Scott Loeliger MD, MS
Director, Mark Stinson
Fellowship in Underserved and
  Global Health
Contra Costa Family Practice
  Residency
Martinez, California

James H. McKerrow, MD, PhD
Director, Sandler Center for
  Drug Discovery
University of California San
  Francisco
San Francisco, California

Gerald Paccione MD
Professor of Clinical Medicine
Albert Einstein College of
  Medicine
Director, Global Health Center
  Education Alliance
Bronx, New York

Suzinne Pak-Gorstein, MD, PhD,
  MPH
Assistant Professor
Department of Pediatrics
University of Washington
Co-Director, Global Health
  Pathway Program
Seattle Children's Hospital
Seattle, Washington

Kathy J. Pedersen, MPAS, RN,
PA-C
Clinical Associate
Adjunct Clinical Faculty
Utah Physician Assistant
  Program
University of Utah School of
  Medicine
Community Health Clinics of
  Salt Lake City
Salt Lake City, Utah

Jeremy Penner, MD
Assistant Clinical Professor
Department of Family Practice
Associate Director, Division of
  Global Health
University of British Columbia
Treasurer, Pamoja
Program Consultant, FACES
Vancouver, British Columbia

Andrea L. Pfeifle, EdD, PT
Director of Education
Department of Family and
  Community Medicine
Director, Center for
  Interprofessional Health Care
University of Kentucky
Lexington, Kentucky

Christopher Prater, MD
Resident Physician
Internal Medicine and Pediatrics
Christiana Health Systems
Wilmington, Delaware

Michael Slatnick, MD
Resident Physician
Department of Family Medicine
University of British Columbia
Vancouver, British Columbia

Nicole St Clair, MD
Assistant Professor of Pediatrics
Medical College of Wisconsin
Director, Department of
  Pediatrics Global Health
  Program
Milwaukee, Wisconsin

Christopher C. Stewart, MD, MA
Associate Professor of Pediatrics
Director, UCSF Global Health
  Pathway to Discovery
University of California San
  Francisco
San Francisco, California

Stephanie Tache, MD
Assistant Professor
Department of Family and
  Community Medicine
Prevention and Public Health
  Group
University of California San
  Francisco
Research Fellow, Institute for
General, Family and Preventative
  Medicine
Paracelsus Medical University
Salzburg, Austria

Flora Teng, MD, MPH
Resident Physician
Department of Obstetrics and
  Gynecology
University of British Columbia
Vancouver, British Columbia

German Tenorio, MD
Regional Medical Director, Child
  Family Health International
Oaxaca, Mexico

Wilfrido Torres, MD
Child Family Health
  International
Quito, Ecuador

Yousef Yassin Turshani, MD
Department of Pediatrics
University of California San
  Francisco
San Francisco, California

Anthony Valdini, MD, MS
Associate Professor in Family
  Medicine and Community
  Health
Tufts University School of
  Medicine
University of Massachusetts
  School of Medicine
Director, Faculty Development
Lawrence Family Medicine
  Residency
Lawrence, Massachusetts

Anvar Velji, MD, FRCP(c),
FACP, FIDSA
Clinical Professor of Medicine
University of California at Davis
Chief of Infectious Diseases
Kaiser Permanente, South
  Sacramento
Co-Founder, Global Health
  Education Consortium
Davis, California

Mary T. White, Ph.D.
Professor and Director, Division
  of Medical Humanities
Boonshoft School of Medicine
Wright State University
Dayton, Ohio

Sophy Shiahua Wong, MD
Assistant Clinical Professor of
  Medicine
University of California San
  Francisco
Attending Physician in Internal
  and HIV Medicine, Asian
  Health Services
HIV Consultant, Pangaea
  Foundation
San Francisco, California

Foreword

Over the past few generations, the rapid growth of transportation and technology has allowed access to previously isolated parts of the world. Enhanced communication is facilitating greater exposure to issues of resource scarcity, especially in the third world. This knowledge has sparked growing humanitarianism and a willingness to help, especially among younger generations. The growing recognition of effects of pollution and environmental degradation, most significantly by industrialized nations, has ignited a new drive toward sustainability and responsible resource utilization. In this new era of focus on equity and sustainability, global health education and training programs are growing in number and influence.

Medical and other health science students learn in new and different ways when working in communities abroad. Visiting trainees observe, see, hear and feel in a vivid way through experience in foreign settings. Unfamiliar cultural and linguistic dimensions, often experienced through service work, spark curiosity and observations that can compliment lessons learned in home communities. These experiences can be challenging, difficult extensions of a learner's comfort zone, testing the flexibility of one's personality and the openness of mind and heart. Such challenges can also lead to new-found independence and confidence, as learners overcome language barriers, begin to understand unfamiliar customs and traditions, and foster connection with local community members over a common goal: Good health for all.

Upon returning to home communities, learners may realize a longer lasting effect of their experience -- the acquisition of new tools to better serve their local populations as professional practitioners.

Those of us privileged with the experience of mentoring international students are enriched by teaching as part of our medical practice. Prior to my involvement with the California-based NGO Child Family Health International (CFHI,) I lacked a strong interest in public health issues and global health programs. Now, through mentoring international students, I have gained exposure to global and public health issues *and* a wider perspective of our own local strengths and weaknesses.

The number of global health areas in need of improvement are manifold: child and adolescent health; women's health; care for those with special needs; geriatrics; elimination of gender, sexuality, and race discrimination in health care; lack of infrastructure and social organization in resource-limited settings. Our recognition of these inequities and our increasing interconnectedness drives the new focus on developing global health programs in academic, governmental and non-profit settings. Program development is a challenge, as every student is different, every cultural setting unique and complex, and the fabric of each community equally vulnerable to the ripples of politics, conflict, and economy.

This 2nd edition, edited by Dr. Evert and Dr. Chase, touches broadly on the many challenges in global health program development. This new version delves deeply into issues of cross-cultural ethics, provides updated information on existing training programs, explores visiting student and host perspectives on exchange and service learning, and examines multiple types of training program models in order to help guide readers to understand the complexity of the growing field of global health education.

Readers will find this text to be an excellent source of information in global health training and program design. Let us continue to pursue this exciting educational task: to select, send, mentor, and bring back great students, to make their international experiences unforgettable and to help shape their learning as health professionals.

Dr. German Tenorio
Regional Medical Director
Child Family Health International
Oaxaca, Mexico

Foreword

The enthusiasm among medical students and residents to participate in global health activities has grown to unprecedented levels. This young entrepreneurial generation has embraced global health as the intersection of their noble interests in both humanitarianism and globalization. They have been asking their medical schools and residency programs for more opportunities to serve resource-poor communities, both in their local neighborhoods as well as distant exotic locales, and have oftentimes created new programs for themselves and others.

Currently, according to recent American Association of Medical Colleges data, nearly one out of every three medical school graduates has participated in global health activities. Yet, nearly two-thirds of those entering the medical profession had planned to participate in global health education or service. The imbalance between those wanting and gaining international experience is even greater among resident physicians, in part due to busier work schedules and fewer structured opportunities. Those who are fortunate enough to participate in international educational activities during their medical training become better physicians for having done so.

Medical schools and residency programs have been struggling to keep up with the global health demands of medical students and residents. Although the number of international programs has been growing steadily over the last several decades, many schools and programs have not had the necessary tools to develop adequate training programs in global health. Dr. Evert and her colleagues at the Global Health Education Consortium have compiled the most practical and useful information for schools and programs to create appropriate global health training opportunities.

The risks of creating global health opportunities that are not culturally or ethically appropriate are profound, and there are abundant stories of cavalier students and residents practicing well beyond their scope of training. In this regard, Drs. Evert, Chase and their colleagues provide an extremely important chapter on ethical considerations in global health. They offer valuable tools to help ensure that medical students and residents operate within their limits and with respect to resource-poor communities. The consequences of unethical practice in international settings could not only bring undue harm to patients, but might also scar the reputation of the global health community at large.

Finally, medical education and residency training may be at the precipice of another major transformational change. As educators are increasingly incorporating more cultural and ethical training, future programs will undoubtedly incorporate a much stronger focus on global health. During this evolutionary process, this book will continue to serve as the definitive guide for developing training programs in global health.

Paul K. Drain, MD, MPH
Fellow, Infectious Diseases
Massachusetts General Hospital
The Brigham and Women's Hospital
Harvard Medical School
Co-author, <u>Caring for the World: A Guidebook to Global Health and Medicine</u>
Boston, Massachusetts

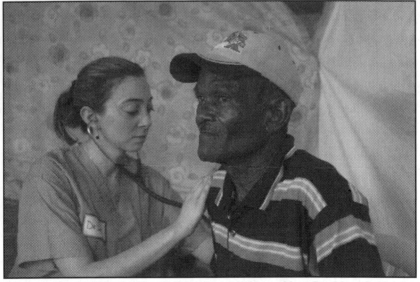

Advocate Christ (Illinois) Hospital family medicine resident Dr. Lissa Goldstein listens to Soto Martinez's lungs in a Health Horizons International Clinic in Negro Melo, Dominican Republic. (Photo credit: Rachel Geylin.)

Introduction to Global Health Education 1

Melanie Anspacher, Jessica Evert and Jerry Paccione

> *The quest to improve global health represents a challenge
> of monumental proportions: the problems seem so
> enormous, the obstacles so great, and success so elusive.
> On the other hand it is difficult to imagine a pursuit more
> closely aligned with the professional values and visceral
> instincts of most physicians. Many young doctors enter
> medicine with a passionate interest in global health; our
> challenge is to nurture this commitment and encourage its
> expression.[1]*

Shaywitz and Ausiello (2002)

Globalization is influencing all sectors of society, including health and
wellness. The preceding quote by *Shaywitz and Ausiello* reflects a growing
body of literature which demonstrates the desire of residency applicants to
engage in global health education during their post-graduate training.[2] In
order to meet this demand, medical residencies are grappling with the
challenges of establishing and expanding global health programming. Since
the 1st edition of this guide book, many programs have incorporated new
and expanded global health education opportunities, however many
challenges remain. Many residencies and institutions experience unique
challenges based on size, level of administrative support, resources, and
other factors. International and field-based experiences during training are
accompanied by ethical questions and dilemmas about sustainability and
impact. As programs seek to incorporate clinical training in new and
unfamiliar settings, they must be aware of the many intended and
unintended consequences of involvement by medical trainees from outside
the host community. These are critical considerations as we prepare the
next generation of a healthcare workforce to care for the communities of the
world.

As a sign of the advancing interest in global health education,
many primary care and specialty societies have established international
subcommittees and seminars, such as the annual *International Family
Medicine Development Workshop* and the *Section on International Child
Health of the American Academy of Pediatrics*. Larger, multidisciplinary
organizations serve to link educators, clinicians and researchers in the effort
to improve communication, training, educational resources, and service in
communities around the world. Such is the mission of the Global Health
Education Consortium (GHEC), which sponsors this text. Concurrent
growth and specialization is happening within the academic sector. A new
sister organization, Consortium of Universities in Global Health (CUGH) is

a membership organization for universities who seek to develop a multi-disciplinary approach across universities to improve global health research, education, and service. Outside of the academic setting, the past decade has also witnessed an increase in the number of non-profit organizations dedicated to global health exposure for future physicians, which include *Child and Family Health International*, *Doctors for Global Health*, and *Community for Children* are a few examples. Many non-profit and non-governmental organizations devoted to improving global health access have also produced educational resources to help both training physicians in highly resourced nations, as well as health care workers in under-resourced communities – these include *Doctors without Borders/Médecins sans Frontiéres*, and the *Bill and Melinda Gates Foundation* among many others.

This remains an exciting time for global health program development. As with any program introduction or expansion, the challenges are manifold. This guidebook attempts to navigate the maze of global health education, provide examples of global health residency training, and identify resources for developing and improving programs, while defining competencies for residents and examining ethical dilemmas of these efforts.

History of the Globalization of Health

Despite the longstanding recognition that medicine and health transcend geographic boundaries, integration of this idea into U.S. medical education and practice has been slow. The field of international health or "global health" – now renamed to emphasize universality and connectedness – has evolved considerably over the last 150 years. During this evolution, the scope and even the definition of the field has been shaped by dynamic tension between interests of patients (clinical) and populations (public health), and within public health, between "vertical" disease-oriented and "horizontal" system-oriented perspectives.

The modern era of "international health" may begin with worldwide cholera epidemic of the mid-1800s. This crisis prompted physicians and politicians to convene the first *International Sanitary Conference* in 1851. For the remainder of the 19th century, successive conferences focused on the most pressing issues in infectious disease, such as yellow fever or bubonic plague. These annual conferences took place until 1938, and evolved into a forum to present and disseminate the newest discoveries in medicine.

In 1902, a hemispheric collaboration to fight yellow fever led to the creation of the *Pan American Sanitary Bureau* (now the *Pan American Health Organization*), which became a model for transnational collaboration for health promotion. Following World War I, international health organizations led by the League of Nations Health Committee broadened their focus from clinical infectious disease to public health issues such as nutrition, and maternal and infant health. Two decades later, the horror of the Holocaust and concentration camps during World War II led to unprecedented international humanitarian cooperation.

In 1947, physicians from 27 countries met in Paris and created the World Medical Association, whose objective is "to serve humanity by endeavoring to achieve the highest international standards in Medical Education, Medical Science, Medical Art and Medical Ethics, and Health Care for all people in the world." The following year, the United Nations created the World Health Organization (WHO) -- a single global entity charged with fostering collaboration among member nations toward a new definition of health: "not merely the absence of disease but the promotion, attainment, and maintenance of physical, mental, and social well-being."

The excitement generated by the WHO's success in eradicating smallpox was soon followed by the failure to eradicate malaria, an effort that exposed the complex interrelationships between health and infrastructure, culture, politics and economic stability. This failure also demonstrated the importance of culturally-sensitive programming, and dispelled the notion of a formulaic clinical approach to complex global health problems. The importance of addressing sociopolitical determinants of health led to the foundation of the non-governmental health organization *Médecins Sans Frontières* (*MSF*, *Doctors Without Borders*.) MSF was founded in 1971 by French physicians dissatisfied with the efforts of WHO and International Red Cross in confronting the structural and political roots of the crisis in Biafra during the Nigerian Civil War. In 1977, at Alma Ata, the WHO declared a shift from disease-specific strategies to primary care and system-based solutions to attain "health for all".

Today, we are increasingly aware that health is determined by a host of biological and social factors, and consequently it depends on partnerships between diverse nations, disciplines and institutions. The economic, human, and environmental consequences of health disparities between populations are being brought to light. Failure of rich and poor countries to work together to diminish these disparities will have disastrous consequences for all. In 2001, the *WHO Macroeconomic Commission on Health* put forth three core findings:

1. The massive amount of disease burden in the world's poorest nations poses a huge threat to global wealth and security.

2. Millions of impoverished people around the world die of preventable and treatable infectious diseases because they lack access to basic medical care and sanitation.

3. We have the potential to save millions of lives each year, but only if the wealthy nations would provide the poorer ones with the requisite services and support.[3]

In order to fulfill in the promise of the WHO commission's third statement, there must be appropriate global health training for professionals in diverse disciplines. In 1948, the first *Student International Clinical Conference* brought together medical students throughout Europe. In 1951, this conference became the *International Federation of Medical Students' Associations*, and defined its objective of "studying and promoting the interests of medical student co-operation on a purely professional basis, and promoting activities in the field of student health and student relief". Its mission soon expanded to include medical student cooperation in improving the health of all populations.

In the U.S., the *International Health Medical Education Consortium* (now called the *Global Health Education Consortium*, *GHEC*), was created in 1991. With a mission to address health disparities through education, and to foster global health education for medical students, GHEC now has a membership of over 90 health professional schools in the U.S.A. and Canada. In addition, the *American Medical Association* opened its *Office of International Medicine* in 1978, the *Global Health Action Committee* of the *American Medical Student Association* was initiated in 1997, and the U.S.A. chapter of *International Federation of Medical Students' Association* (IFMSA) was inaugurated in 1998. Today, many professional specialty organizations have their own global health committees.

Indeed in this age of globalization, professional and technical personnel from non-medical fields such as law, business, and engineering are joining forces to meet the multifaceted challenges to world health. Along with medical faculty, educators in these diverse fields are working to identify skill sets necessary for collaborative global health work, and to cultivate the passion for this work among their trainees. Recently, the Lancet published the report "Health professionals for a new century: transforming education to strengthen health systems in an interdependent world."[4] This report is an indictment of the current shortfalls in the medical education system that are perpetuating health inequities at home and abroad by not keeping pace with the challenges of modern healthcare including globalization, distribution of resources, and cost-responsive care. The commission behind this report proposes an overhaul of medical and health education to adopt a global, multi-disciplinary systems-based approach. The report provides further support for the momentum witnessed in incorporating global health into graduate medical education.

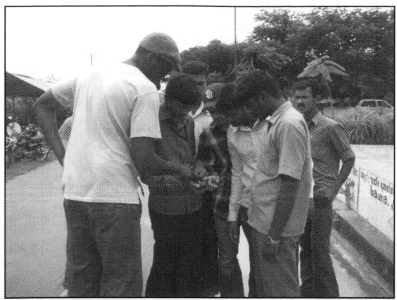

Ben Thomas (UCSF School of Medicine) and Miguel Pinedo (UC Berkeley, School of Public Health) of the UCSF Global Health Frameworks Program train staff at Swami Vivekananda Youth Movement in Saragur, India to use GPS technology. (Photo credit: K. Holbrook.)

Literature Review of Global Health Graduate Medical Education

An article in the November 1969 issue of the Journal of the American Medical Association reported, "every U.S.A. medical school is involved in such international activities as faculty travel for study, research and teaching, clinical training for foreign graduates, and medical student study overseas...a recent self-survey by Case Western Reserve medical students indicated that 78% of the first-year class and 85% of the second-year class were interested in studying or working abroad at sometime in their medical school careers."[5] The article went on to report that 600 American medical students went abroad during the academic year 1966-1967.

This interest in global health continues today, although the progress that one might anticipate in 40 years toward integration of global health into undergraduate and graduate medical education is slow. Results of recent surveys by the Association of American Medical Colleges show that the proportion of American medical students taking an international elective during medical school has increased significantly over the last decade, from under 15% in 1998 to almost 30% in 2006.[6] More and more medical schools have begun offering formal training in global health. As opportunities for training increase, it is likely that demand for continued and more specialized training during residency will follow. A recent survey of surgical residents indicated 98% were interested in an international elective

5

and 73% would prioritize it over any other elective.[7] Similarly, a study of primary care residents from various disciplines demonstrated 58% were interested in global health.[8] However, out of the residents surveyed, only 8% had participated in an international elective. Among that small group, 82% planned to continue to work in global health and 100% expressed an ongoing dedication to underserved populations domestically. These findings demonstrate the unmet needs for global health education and immersion experiences. In addition, it appears that these activities may inspire, or at least propel, a dedication to further global health work and service to impoverished populations domestically.

Availability of Global Health Training

Most specialties have gathered, or are in the process of gathering, data on the availability of international training in their disciplines. These data show rising interest in global health education, and efforts by training institutions to provide such education. A recent study among pediatric training institutions found that 59% of programs offered global health training, while 21% of residents participated in such training. Characteristics associated with participating in global health training included being single (p<.01), younger (p<.05), without children (p<.01), have less educational debt (<.05), larger residency program (p<.001) Tellingly, less than half of residents who were definitely or likely to take part in global health activities after graduation, received training in a majority of content areas considered necessary for such work.[9] A recent cross-sectional survey of all pediatric residency programs accredited by the Accreditation Council for Graduate Medical Education (ACGME) revealed a substantial increase in availability of global health electives.[10] Of the programs that responded (53%), over half had offered a global health elective in the preceding year, and 47% had incorporated global health education into their residency curricula. Programs reported providing support to residents in various ways, including faculty mentorship, clinical training and orientation, post-elective debriefing, and funding.

Within family medicine, a 1998 survey found that 54% of programs offered global health training, while 15% of programs offered curricular and financial support for such training. Logistic regression analysis of these data suggested that the longevity of the global health programming, covering of living expenses at the international site, and involvement of faculty in international work in the past two years were correlated with increased likelihood of participation of residents in global health activities.[11]

A 2007 survey of U.S. surgical residents found that 98% were interested in international electives even though global health electives and programs are limited within surgical programs.[12] Although no surveys have been published in the realm of orthopedic surgery, the University of

California, San Francisco, orthopedic surgery residency reports 41% its residents took part in international electives, prompting it to establish a longitudinal program with Orthopedics Overseas in Umtata, South Africa.[13]

In addition to primary and surgical programs with strong dedication to global health education, the field of emergency medicine has distinguished itself through the establishment of global health fellowships. In their 2005 article, Anderson and Aschkenasy discuss goals of recently established international emergency medicine fellowships: (1) To develop the ability to assess international health systems and identify pertinent emergency health issues; (2) To design emergency health programs that address identified needs; (3) To develop the skills necessary to implement emergency programs abroad and integrate them into existing health systems; and (4) To develop the ability to evaluate the quality and effectiveness of international health programs.[14]

Effect of International Rotations on Participants

Efforts have been made to investigate the benefits of international electives to medical students and residents. In a study of medical students and residents who participated in international health electives, attitudes toward the importance of doctor-patient communication, use of symbolism by patients, public health interventions, and community health programs were more positive after than before their experience. When participants were re-interviewed 2 years later, a statistically significant proportion reported continued positive influences from the experience on their clinical and language skills, sensitivity to cultural and socioeconomic factors, awareness of the role of communication in clinical care, and attitudes toward careers working with the underserved (p<.01).[15] A similar positive impact on self-assessed cultural competence and sense of idealism was found in a study of clinical medical students who had completed an international elective.[16] In comparison with students who did not choose an international elective, students with international experience showed significantly higher levels of idealism, enthusiasm, and interest in primary care, as well as sharpened perception of the need to understand cultural differences.

Studies of medical students participating in international electives indicate improvements on standardized tests, as well as subjective knowledge acquisition. One study showed that medical students who participated in a 3-6-week international program scored significantly higher in the preventive medicine/public health sections of the USMLE board exam than a control group.[17] In another study, medical student participants said their international experience sharpened awareness of the importance of public health and patient education.[18] Seventy-eight percent of the students also reported a heightened awareness of cost issues and financial barriers to patient care. All students in this group also reported that they had a greater appreciation of the history and physical exam as diagnostic tests.

7

Similar effects have been found for medical residents receiving international health training or completing an elective. Data and commentary have been published on residents in a variety of fields including internal medicine[19,20,21], surgery[22], multi-disciplinary programs[23], neurology[24], and pediatrics[25]. An evaluation of 162 multi-disciplinary residents who undertook an international rotation indicated the experience led to increased exposure to an array of pathology, increased understanding of working with limited resources, improvement in surgical or clinical skills, and increased interactions with novel cultures.[23] Participants in an international health program in internal medicine were more likely than non-participants to believe that U.S. physicians underused their physical exam and history-taking skills and reported that the experience had a positive influence on their clinical diagnostic skills.[19] An internal medicine elective program was found to have a positive impact on tropical medicine knowledge for participants.[20] Participants in a pediatric international health elective reported seeing a significant number of diseases and clinical presentations that they had never encountered at their home institution.[25] Notably missing from the current literature is an evaluation of the impacts residents have on their international hosts.

With regard to particular competency-based knowledge acquisition, Anspacher et al. surveyed graduating pediatric residents. By self-report, residents who achieved education or training relevant to specific global health topics was varied.

Percentages of Graduating Pediatric Residents Achieving Specific Global Health Education Objectives, from a Self-Report Survey[9]	
Health care of immigrant or refugee children and their families	54%
Diagnosis and management of common pediatric tropical disease	49%
epidemiology of infant and child mortality in developing countries	44%
preparation for work or volunteer experience in a developing country	32%
Ethical issues in working or volunteering in developing countries	27%
International child health policies, initiatives, and guidelines	25%
Preparation for responding to humanitarian emergencies	22%

Similar data across other groups of trainees is limited. Competency specific training goals are described in Chapter 4: Competency-Based Global Health Education, and assessment of these goals in Global Health Program Evaluation in Chapter 6.

Impact of Global Health Education on Residency Training and Career Path

International health opportunities appear to play a role in applicants' ranking of residency programs. At a pediatric residency program in

Colorado where a formal international health elective is offered, 67% of residents cited the opportunity as a major factor in ranking the program.[25] Similarly, 42% of residents surveyed at Duke University's Internal Medicine Residency Program cited their well-established International Health Program as a significant factor in ranking.[20] In 1993, at the University of Cincinnati Family Medicine Residency Program, an official International Health Track was implemented through which residents were able to complete an international elective and receive year-round didactic training. A survey of the program graduates from 1994 to 2003 found that participants in the International Health Track ranked it as the most important factor in choosing the program. Residents in the track were more likely to have relocated farther from both their medical school and home city for residency than non-participants, indicating the appeal of the track. Although the pool of medical students from US medical schools applying to family medicine programs had been declining in the 1990s, during the years following implementation of this program, match rates for the program improved from 70% to 100.[26] This study supports the dual benefits of such education on both medical trainees and training programs.

Larger surveys in specific specialties also demonstrate the interest in global health training. A survey of first year emergency medicine residents in the United States in 2001, found that 62% of respondents who had interviewed at programs with international opportunities considered this a positive factor in the ranking process, 58% perceived the need for additional training in an international setting, and 76% indicated a desire for increased international EM exposure in their current residency program.[27] In family medicine, the presence of an international health track has been demonstrated to influence the residency selection process and is seen as a means of recruitment.[29] In their survey of graduating pediatric residents, Anspacher et al. found that 22% considered global health training essential/very important when choosing a residency, while 36% considered it somewhat important.[9]

Global health education and international experiences appear to also affect choices about future practice environment or specialty. Medical students who participated in an international health experience in a developing country were more likely later to practice in underserved areas in the U.S.A.[28] During 1995-1997, 60 senior medical students were chosen to participate in the International Health Fellowship, an intensive two week course followed by a two month rotation in an underserved country. When participants were surveyed several years after completing the fellowship, most of them reported it had significantly influenced their careers. The majority of respondents were practicing primary care, and over half had participated in community health projects or had done further work overseas.[29] Internal medicine residents who participated in international electives were found more likely to change career plans from subspecialty to general medicine[19] or public health.[20] International health experience in

9

training and future practice in primary care, public health, or in underserved communities appears consistently associated across studies.

Following residency training, there are many potential barriers to long term commitment by U.S. trained physicians in international communities. Medical school debt may be one such issue. An International Health Service Corps has been proposed, through which physicians would provide clinical care and capacity-building in developing countries in exchange for educational debt forgiveness.[30] This and other efforts to make global service careers more feasible for US physicians are necessary.

Program Development and Challenges

A variety of disciplines have published work on program design and development challenges. Program intensity and curricular content varies greatly. For example, the Howard Hiatt Residency in Global Health Equity and Internal Medicine based at Brigham and Women's Hospital provides a four-year training program that includes customary internal medicine training, augmented by didactic teaching, longitudinal seminars, international research project, and structured mentoring (see also, Chapter 10: Profiles of Global Health Programs.) The program trains physicians to develop community-based health care skills and to advocate for and research health disparities both domestically and internationally. Development of the program involved recruitment of faculty with experience in caring for underserved populations and with an interest in health care disparities. These faculty members provide strong mentorship for residents – a strength of the program. The core competencies of the Howard Hiatt Residency in Global Health Equity and Internal Medicine are as follows:

1. Evaluate and address the social determinants of health and disease.
2. Acquire clinical skills necessary to take care of patients with a wide range of health problems in resource-poor settings.
3. Conduct research relating to health disparities and global health.
4. Attain skills in advocacy, leadership, and operational management of global health programs.
5. Obtain in-depth knowledge about the specific public health and medical problems affecting one geographic region of the world.
6. Develop a strong base in the ethics of international medical practice and research.
7. Master language fluency to practice medicine, conduct public advocacy and carry out research in a geographic area of interest.

Importantly, the competencies of the Howard Hiatt program require residents to choose a geographic focus and develop multi-pronged competencies (including language, research, advocacy, and clinical skills). This program is unique in the comprehensiveness, geographic focus, and linkage of domestic and global health disparities. The 3 year program follows a standard internal medicine internship.[31]

While the Howard Hiatt program offers a unique 4 year curriculum in global health and disparities, this program is only available to 2 residents per year and requires significant financial and personnel resources. This program offers exceptional training. Other approaches described in the literature may be more feasible when resources and institutional support is limited.

University of California, San Francisco's Department of Surgery has published a descriptive article on the pilot of a 6-week clinical surgical elective. Reacting to great interest on behalf of surgical residents (90% expressed interest in a developing an in-country elective outside the United States), and building on an existing university relationship with Makerere University in Kampala and an existing internal medicine rotation at the same site, a surgical rotation was created. The creation of this program demonstrates the impact of university-wide momentum (driven by the UCSF Global Health Sciences department,) in partnership with existing relationships with international sites. For UCSF surgical residents, this momentum has opened doors for novel rotations and programming.[32] A follow-up evaluation of the UCSF surgical elective program over a 5 year period demonstrated effective integration of the elective into an academic surgical residency program. Many involved residents also pursued advanced degrees in public health and undertook a multi-disciplinary global health training track. The authors also note the need for reciprocity for the host institution. In this case, host physicians and trainees collaborated with visiting faculty and residents in research projects. Thus far, there are no studies which have reviewed the success and adequacy of reciprocity as perceived by host institutions or individuals.

Individuals and institutions in many disciplines of medicine have published specialty-specific research on program development. In 2007, Evert and colleagues presented resources for faculty and curriculum development in "Going Global: Considerations for Introducing Global Health into Family Medicine Programs."[33] Such discussions are especially important for programs with limited internal resources who are interested in global health curriculum development.

While most longstanding international elective experiences are funded and supported by residency and fellowship programs and other institutions, a large number of residents go abroad as individuals, without established institutional or formal host community relationships. Such individually organized experiences often involve partnerships between trainees and individual physicians on short-term mission or volunteer experiences. The merits of such activities can be debated from multiple perspectives, but the existence of such activities is important to acknowledge. A documented example is described by Jarman et al. in the Journal of Surgical Education.[34] A PGY-3 surgical resident accompanied a cardiothoracic and general surgeon with significant international experience on a 2-week elective. The goals of the program were to provide surgical experience in a rural, underserved, international setting and to instill an appreciation of volunteer service in the resident. The attending surgeon was board certified by the American Board of Surgery, and the rotation offered a global health short-term mission experience. Interaction and collaboration with host country general surgeons was an important component of the experience. The surgical resident participated in 63 surgical procedures, some of which for the first time in his career, over a 9 day period. The residency program accepted this rotation for credit, based on fulfillment of appropriate ACGME core competencies.

The outcomes of all types of away experiences, both individual and institutionally-organized, and short versus long-term, should be evaluated and impacts assessed by involved trainees *and* supervising educators. In order to promote responsible global health involvement, we must all be aware of our impact, most importantly on those we serve – the host community and individuals, as well as host institutions. Framework for program evaluation and a discussion on global health ethics are found in Chapters 3 and 6.

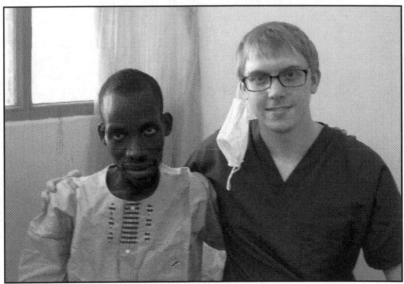

Thomas Quinn, first year student at Albert Einstein College of Medicine, and Mr. O, a Senegalese patient, at Centre Hospitalier National Universitaire de Fann in Dakar, Senegal. (Photo credit: Christina Tan)

Barriers to Training

Establishing global health curricula in residency programs presents numerous challenges. As with all development, locating financial support is a main constraint. Sustainability – program, partnerships, faculty, and institutional support – is critical to ongoing success. The field of global health is largely supported, at present, by educational institutions and by a combination of private and federal funding (medical schools and universities, Partners in Health, and PEPFAR are respective examples.) Funding streams can change year to year and are vulnerable to changes in economic and political priorities. International partners are vulnerable to changes in home country support and new challenges to public health.[35]

A specific financial barrier to global health graduate medical education is the potential loss of funding authorized by the Center for Medicare and Medicaid Services for residents rotating abroad. In order to solve this issue, some programs recruit a greater number than the quota of residents that the federal system will support, allowing "extra" residents for a given time period to rotate at sites that may not fulfill CMS requirements, both in domestic and international settings. Funding these extra residents is an issue, and residencies must find other funding streams to support extra resident positions, from academic, hospital and grant-based sources.

Fulfillment of curricular requirements set by ACGME and specialty boards is another critical step. An increasing set of resources for competency-based global health education are available, with specific application to different disciplines of medicine. Chapters 2, 4 and 5 review curriculum development, competency-based education and program considerations.

Controversies

As the base of global health literature develops and published dialogues become more frequent, a variety of challenges and controversies come to light. At a very basic level, we must be introspective and honest about our goals, the cost and alternatives to our current path in global health education, and the stakeholders and beneficiaries of this work. In response to Drain and colleagues' article,[35] Dr. Chandrakanth Are, a surgeon and educator at the University of Nebraska with training in multiple international sites including the UK and India, raises legitimate questions about the motivations of western residents and programs.[36] He asserts that patients in developing countries are being used as extensions of US graduate medical education and should be recognized as such. Dr. Are highlights the need for screening of candidates for international rotations, emphasizing the requirements of a health diplomat- including comprehension of the educational, ethical, moral, and altruistic implications of global health engagement.

Experiences in global communities are rich with meaning and full of complex questions. Global health is an expansive field including government, industry, non-profit and educational institutions, affecting billions of people and using billions of dollars of resources yearly. For trainees interested in working in host communities with underserved patients, the details of a given trip can be overwhelming – itineraries, supply lists, knowledge base, language training, curriculum requirements – not to mention the larger context. In order to build an ethical foundation among trainees, global health education should include open discussion about the many factors, philosophical and ethical, financial and geopolitical, and personal, individual motivations which shape global health work. The role and time for altruism and ethical education is not standardized.

One example of global health education with an emphasis on ethical involvement can be found at Child Family Health International (CFHI), a non-governmental organization which facilitates global health education for health sciences students. CFHI, whose motto is "Let the world change you," strives to place health sciences students in host communities, so that they may learn about community health care and public health, gain cultural and language competency, and build personal skills while respecting local cultural and ethical boundaries. The goals of this education are manifold, including developing participants' interest in future work in underserved settings. CFHI and its local partners provide the opportunity for this education and exploration without placing students in roles of inappropriate responsibility – a problem which can arise when motivated trainees are placed in communities with tremendous need and lack of oversight or guidance. In addition to guidance and mentorship in its rotations, CFHI also promotes the importance of altruism, helping students to recognize that "activities to serve others are a form of self-fulfillment and enlightened self interest."[37] The meaning of this type of experiential education in global settings is demonstrated in Sawatsky et al.'s survey of residents in the Mayo International Health Program. One resident commented, "more important than their diseases were the patients themselves. The patients introduced me to a culture that, despite extreme poverty, is enriched by strong family values and a sense of community. I was impressed with how willing and eager people were to help each other. I have never met patients so gracious, so in need, as these. It was extremely gratifying to administer health care to this community."[23]

While current articles have reviewed the benefits of global health exposure for residents, there have been no studies on the effects of residents on host communities, institutions and local health care provision. Effects on host communities by visiting medical trainees are undoubtedly complex. Pertinent questions include:

- *How is the availability of services at the host clinical site affected by visiting residents? (Does the extra work capacity offset the need for language and cultural interpretation, time spent by staff in*

14

orientation and supervision of visitors, and loss of work time by local and visiting physicians in order to provide oversight for trainees?)

- *How do international medical education partnerships affect host country institutions? What are the determinants of success and advancement for host country institutions?*
- *How does the overall quality of care for host community members change with the addition of international visiting trainees?*
- *What is the balance of cost and return of services for communities and institutions which host visiting residents?*

Research about these questions from the host perspective is lacking. As a comparison, in the US health care system, residents enhance access for clinical services, usually in hospitals and outpatient clinics which serve a significant number of patients with state and federal health insurance (Medicare and Medicaid.) Despite increasing access to services, residency education results in a net cost when support structures, teachers, and supervising clinicians are considered. The cost of residency training in the United States is subsidized by the Centers for Medicare and Medicaid Services (CMS,) and the resulting balance provides acceptable benefits for all stakeholders. This balance of costs and benefits does not necessarily occur in international settings.

Resident education in visiting rotations requires significant resources, including support staff time, translation services, nursing, attending physician, facility fees, food/housing costs and many others – these costs are incurred, at least in part, by host facilities and institutions. Ozgediz et al. recommend reciprocity between United States residency programs and host partners via visiting faculty from the United States and collaborative research opportunities for host country clinicians.[32] While large academic medical centers in the USA may be able to provide this reciprocity, smaller schools and non-profits may need to develop other means to compensate host institutions. Compensation for teaching and accommodation of visiting residents by local providers and communities is an essential consideration for any global health education program. In the coming years, we need to examine more closely who's benefitting from our global health engagement and ensure true reciprocity with host communities, institutions, and colleagues. Further discussion about building effective partnerships is found in subsequent chapters (Chapter 3 on ethical framework, Chapter 5 on program development, and Chapter 6 on program evaluation.)

Next Steps

The field of global health work is changing. United States' involvement in international health work began over 150 years ago as a response by physicians and politicians to infectious disease pandemics in mostly distant, under-resourced settings. The field of global health has since evolved to an ever expanding network of allied health professionals and associated colleagues, who recognize many new and persistent challenges to global wellness – environmental degradation, chronic disease, armed conflict, resource scarcity, discrimination and racism, and socio-economic determinants of health. The field has become a more inclusive, overarching framework of individuals and organizations from many professional disciplines and many countries. We recognize that the underlying challenges to health and wellness in our own communities are increasingly similar to those in other nations.

This text highlights the importance of basic global health education to medical students, residents, and allied health professionals; and provides a guide on how to initiate, develop and sustain ethical, reciprocal and meaningful global health education. The realities of poverty, disease, geopolitical strife, and resource scarcity are unavoidable, and they must be understood and addressed in the effort to improve the standard of health in all communities. The provision of this education is just one small step in the global health commitment we need to make to the world's neediest patients. In addition to making global health education an integrated part of undergraduate and graduate medical education, we need to consider how the U.S. educational system, and the educational systems in similar, highly resourced nations, can contribute to workforce shortages, advocate for underserved patients, and systemically address issues of health inequities in our own backyards and abroad. It is imperative for health within and outside our borders that U.S.-trained health professionals have competency in global health. As the Health Professionals for a New Century report concludes, "globalizing medical education is an imperative, not an option."[4]

References

[1] D Shaywitz and D Ausiello. Global Health: A Chance for Western Physicians to Give and Receive. The American Journal of Medicine. 2002;113(4)354-7.
[2] Thompson MJ, Huntington MK, Hunt DD, Pinsky LE, Brodie JJ. Educational effects of international health electives on US and Canadian medical students and residents: a literature review. Acad Med. 2003;78:342-47.
[3] Macroeconomics and Health: Investing in Health for Economic Development: Report of the Commission on Macroeconomics and Health. Jeffrey D. Sachs, Chair. Presented 20 December 2001.
[4] Frenk J et al. Health Professionals for a new century: transforming education to strengthen health systems in an interdependent world. The Lancet, Early Online Publication, Nov 29 2010, doi:10.1016/S0140-6736(08)61345-8.
[5] International Medical Education. JAMA 1969;210(8):1555-57
[6] Association of American Medical Colleges. 2006 Medical School Graduate Questionnaire. Available at www.aamc.org/data/gq/allschoolreports/2006.pdf. Accessed April 5, 2007.

[7] Powell A et al. International Experience, Electives, and Volunteerism in Surgical Training: A Survey of Resident Interest. J Am Coll Surg; vol 205, July 2007: 162-168.

[8] Bauer T, Sanders J. Needs assessment of Wisconsin primary care residents and faculty regarding interest in global health training. BMC Medical Education, 2009,9:36.

[9] Anspacher et al. National Survey of Pediatric Resident Training in Global Health. Poster Presentation, American Academy of Pediatrics, 2010.

[10] Nelson BD, Lee ACC, Newby PK, Chamberlin MR, Huang C. Global health training in pediatric residency programs. Pediatrics. July 2008; 122(1):28-33.

[11] Schultz SH, Rousseau S. International health training in family practice residency programs. Family Medicine. 1998 Jan; 30(1):29-33

[12] Powell AC, Mueller C, Kingham P. International electives and volunteerism in surgical training: a survey of resident interest. J Am Col Surg. 2007 July;205(1):162-8.

[13] Haskell A, Rovinsky D, Brown HK, Coughlin RR. The UCSF international orthopedic elective. Clin Orthop. 2002 March;396:12-18.

[14] Anderson PD, Aschkenasy M, Lis J. International emergency medicine fellowships. Emerg Med Clin North Am. 2005 Feb;23(1):199-215.

[15] Haq C, Rothenberg D, Gjerde C, et al. "New world views: preparing physicians in training for global health work." Family Medicine 2000;32:566-72.

[16] Godkin MA, Savageau JA. "The Effect of a Global Multiculturalism Track on Cultural Competence of Preclinical Medical Students." Family Medicine. 2001;33(3):178-86.

[17] Waddell WH, Kelley PR, Suter E, Levit EJ. Effectiveness of an international health elective as measured by NBME Part II. J Med Educ. 1976 Jun;51(6):468-72.

[18] Bissonette R, Route C. "The Educational Effect of Clinical Rotations in Nonindustrialized Countries." Family Medicine 1994;26:226-31.

[19] Gupta et al. "The International Health Program: The Fifteen-Year Experience With Yale University's Internal Medicine Residency Program." American Journal of Tropical Medicine and Hygiene 1999;61(6).

[20] Miller WC, Corey GR, Lallinger GJ, Durack DT. International Health and internal medicine residency training: the Duke University experience. Am J Med 1995;99(3):291-7.

[21] Furin et al. A Novel Training Model to Address Health Problems in Poor and Underserved Populations. Journal of Health Care for the Poor and Underserved;17(2006):17-24.

[22] Jayarman et al. Global Health in General Surgery Residency: A National Survey. J Am Coll Surg, March 2009;208(3):426-33.

[23] Sawatsky et al. Eight Years of Mayo International Health Program: What an International Elective Adds to Resident Education. Mayo Clin Proc, August 2010: 85(8):734-41.

[24] Dahodwala N. Neurology education and global health: my rotation in Botswana. Neurology. 2007 Mar; 68(13):E15-6.

[25] Federico, et al. A Successful International Child Health Elective: The University of Colorado's Department of Pediatrics experience. Arch Pediatr Adolesc Med. 2006 Feb;160(2):191-6.

[26] Bazemore AW, Henein M, Goldenhar LM, Szaflarski M, Lindsell CJ, Diller P. The Effect of Offering International Health Training Opportunities on Family Medicine Residency Recruiting. Fam Med. 2007; 39(4):255-60.

[27] Dey CC, Grabowski JG, Gebreyes, et al. Influence of International Emergency Medicine opportunities on Residency Program Selection. Acad Emerg Med. 2002.

[28] Chiller TM, De Mieri P, Cohen I. "International Health Training. The Tulane Experience." Infectious Disease Clinics of North America. 1995;9:439-43.

[29] Ramsey AH, Haq C, Gjerde CL, Rothenberg D. Career influence of an international health experience during medical school. Fam Med. 2004 Jun;36(6):412-6.

[30] Kerry et al. An International Service Corps for Health- An Unconventional Prescription for Diplomacy. NEJM 2010; 363:13, 1199-1201.

[31] Furin et al. A Novel Training Model to Address Health Problems in Poor and Underserved Populations. Journal of Health Care for the Poor and Underserved;17(2006):17-24.

[32] Ozgediz D, Roayaie K, Debas H, Schecter W, Farmer D.Arch Surg. 2005 Aug;140(8):795-800

[33] Evert et al. Going Global: Considerations for Introducing Global Health Into Family Medicine Training Programs. Fam Med 2007;39(9):659-65.

[34] Jarman et al. Development of an International Elective in a General Surgery Residency. Journal of Surgical Education. 66(4)Aug 2009, 222-224.

[35] Drain PK et al. Global health training and international clinical rotations during residency: Current status, needs and opportunities. Acad Med. 2009;84:320-325.

[36] Are, C. Global health training for residents, letter to the editor. Academic Medicine;84(9):Sept 2009, 1171-2.

[37] Evert J, Huish R, Heit G, Jones E, Loeliger S, Schmidbauer S, Global Health Ethics. In J Iles and BJ Sahakian (Eds.), Oxford Hand book of Neuroethics. Oxford, UK, Forthcoming, 2011.

Kevin Chan, Lisa L. Dillabaugh, Andrea L. Pfeifle, Christopher C. Stewart, and Flora Teng

As interest in global health increases among medical students and residents, residency programs are challenged to provide opportunities to expand knowledge and pursue training in this emerging field. Most medical schools are developing global health programs, largely on the basis of resident demand. Admissions departments and program directors are increasingly aware that residents consider global health opportunities in their selection process.[1,2] Given this interest among applicants, global health training will play a key role as residency programs try to attract high-quality candidates.

Global health training in medical education ranges from establishing overseas rotations to developing didactic experiences, and even incorporating Master's degrees or fellowships into the curriculum.[3] Early training programs have been around for decades, while many more are being established in response to increasing resident demand.

Global health education is not limited to those with strong interests in global health careers. It has been shown that trainees who participate in international electives improve their physical exam skills, become more cost conscious, and show greater commitment to underserved populations.[1,3,4] Thus, the resident audience for global health education spans those without any identified interest in international health to those anticipating careers in it. Providing global health education to residents comes in many forms, some of which are outlined below.

Considerations

Time is a critical factor in providing comprehensive global health education during residency. Medical school offers much more opportunity for elective courses and longitudinal experiences, particularly in the first two years. The amount of time available for global health education in residency is restricted by Residency Review Committee (RRC) and ACGME requirements, which limit elective time. Work hour restrictions might make evening conference or seminar sessions difficult and even impossible to require. Programs must be creative in providing opportunities for residents to complete projects, to perform research, or to work abroad. The difficulty in carving out dedicated time has led some programs to consider adding an extra year to residency dedicated in part toward earning a Master's or other graduate degree.

Most comprehensive programs would benefit from creating a mission statement and vision early in the process. These can be guides as a program develops and form the basis for program objectives and evaluation of program outcomes. Examples of objectives and competency-based program guidelines are found in Chapter 4. Once a global health education program has described its mission and vision, it must identify resources and faculty champions to support the delivery and sustainability of the program.[5] Chapter 5 focuses on specifics of global health program integration into a residency environment.

Goals and Objectives of Global Health Education Programs

Goals for global health curricula in resident education programs should be consistent with the mission and vision statements, conceptualized early in the development of the program. One basic goal for a global health residency might be to meet residents' demand for structured and supervised experiential learning opportunities abroad. Specific content to address this goal should include proper supervision, clear expectations for participants, pre-trip preparation and post-trip debriefing, evaluation from both host supervisors and resident participants, and some type of report or presentation about the experience. Print and on-line resources for global health instruction can be found in Chapter 8. Other goals might include the following:

- Coursework and other educational options for concentrated learning within the discipline of global health;
- Mentorship in research, program development and evaluation, and education program development in resource-poor countries; and
- Exposure to research, academic, and other career opportunities in global health.

Objectives should be written to direct resident learning and expressed in relationship to specific competency areas, as appropriate to the global health education program. These might most appropriately include those in the competency areas of systems-based practice and interpersonal communication skills at a minimum, but could easily also include medical knowledge, patient care, practice-based learning and improvement, and/or professionalism. Chapter 4 further discusses core competencies in Global health Education.

What Constitutes a Global Health Curriculum?

As in medical education as a whole, educators in global health are working to develop core competencies as a foundation to training programs. Houpt and colleagues have identified three domains that should be addressed in Global Health curricula – global burden of disease, traveler's medicine, and immigrant health.[2] These domains represent general competencies that are equally relevant in trainees' home communities and abroad. More specific core competencies can be found both for the field generally, as well as within specialties. Surgeons and psychiatrists, for example, might view the focus of global health training quite differently. An example of global health core competencies in pediatrics developed by the American Academy of Pediatrics can be found in Chapter 7.

Curricular Content

In general, global health curricula can include the following structural components: Experiential (i.e., local and global activities), Didactic (i.e., conferences, lectures, article review), and/or Research/Scholarly Work (i.e., community-based projects, participatory research). General content areas for a global health curriculum, then, could include the following: an overview of global health and the global burden of disease; health indicators and an understanding of their use and limitations; economic and social development; institutions and organizations involved in global health, including policy and trade agreements; environmental health, including water acquisition and safety, natural and man-made disasters, and immigration issues; zoonoses; cultural, social and behavioral determinants of health; demography; social justice and global health including an understanding of human rights; personal health and safety during global health field experiences; global health ethics and professionalism, and cultural competency training.

Core content might also include specific diseases or topics such as malaria, tuberculosis, HIV, measles, nutrition, and maternal and child health, considered separately or woven into other subjects. Competencies and skills in global health may be taught in parallel or integrated into existing residency training. Development of excellent clinical skills and broad training in a specialty is central to a residency program and should not be sacrificed in the process of global health experiences. On the contrary, field experiences may help to promote skills that are underutilized in more-highly resourced settings. Additionally, skills in leadership, program management, and program evaluation are key competencies shared by resident training programs and global health education, thus allowing for joint emphasis.

Laboratory skills might also be taught, with a review of gram stains, malaria preps, and other procedures often referred to specialists or technicians in affluent countries. Basic radiology competence, even physical exam skills, might be included, as many residents in under-resourced settings may be required to rely on their own capabilities to arrive at a diagnosis.

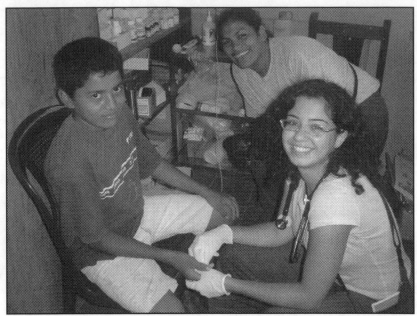

Negar Aliabadi, MD (Tufts University medical student at the time of this photo) and Myriam Salazar, NGO Bridges to Community health worker, with a patient during a clinic visit in Tadazna, RAAN, Nicaragua. (Photo credit: Kristin Anderson.)

Teaching Methods

While the transition from medical school to residency changes the focus of medical education from didactic to clinical training, lectures still provide a strong base for learning core information in post-graduate education. Didactics with a global health focus can be integrated into regular resident conferences and grand rounds. Similarly, journal clubs reviewing historically important, current, or controversial global health topics provide valuable opportunities for residents to gain knowledge. Many institutions also have global health interest groups that hold evening lectures, providing residents with both didactic material and the opportunity to network with faculty and community practitioners working in global health.

On-line teaching modules are excellent venues to learn core concepts and skills and are becoming more popular. The *Global Health Education Consortium* (*GHEC*) has a series of over 80 modules that span topics from zoonoses & vector-borne diseases to social marketing in Asia. These modules are available free on the web and can be used for individual study or as supplement to an instructor-led global health course.[6] More examples on-line material are presented in Chapter 8. Video-taped lectures are now available, and likely will increase in number with the application of technology to medical education. Ensuring that residents absorb and can apply this material can be more challenging, although some on-line lessons have pre- and post-tests that instructors can use to stimulate more engaged participation.

Another teaching model takes advantage of the rotation-based structure used by most residency programs to devote up to a month to global health in lieu of an elective rotation. This affords committed residents the time to dedicate their energy to learning about global health, develop projects or research, and plan their careers. As mentioned, some programs offer an expanded residency option in global health with an extra year, which allows didactic time to be incorporated in a more concentrated format. The University of British Columbia in Canada has combined both of these options into a 6-month program for Enhanced Skills in Global Health. This course is available for Family Medicine residents following their 2-years of core training.[7] The introduction to the program takes place at a one month global health course offered by the University of Arizona,[8] followed by 4 weeks of a tropical medicine elective and 9 weeks of didactic teaching at the University of British Columbia on topics from HIV/AIDS to epidemiology. The capstone for the course is an 8 week field study. Lastly, residents are encouraged to enter into a 6-12 month international commitment following the program.

International Immersion Experiences

Many residency programs support travel to developing countries for short periods during training. In order to follow the residency calendar, these experiences are often a month-long visit to an established site in collaboration with the resident's home institution. The strongest formalized international health electives identify mentors abroad and at home, prepare residents with pre-departure orientation, and focus on collaboration with sites where visiting residents can contribute meaningfully to the host institution or organization. Trainees that have been a part of this type of program report significantly greater impact on their education and career paths as compared to isolated immersion experiences.[4] Through faculty mentorship, pre-departure training, and debriefing after the experience, residents have greater clarity, accountability, and opportunities to meet their learning objectives.[9]

Trainees with particular interests and ingenuity may also pursue electives independently through various means, including working with faculty mentors with overseas connections, contacting universities and hospitals directly, or getting involved with non-governmental organizations. Although these electives allow residents to tailor experiences to their interests, they can be complicated by uncertain mentorship and supervision in host communities. Some programs allow residents to take a leave of absence from training or are flexible enough for residents to take several months or more off for international health research or projects. Projects of this magnitude often require residents to obtain funding and direct their projects themselves. Issues related to funding for resident international experiences are covered in Chapter 5.

Exchanges

If the goals or mission statement of a global health program include helping improve conditions for international partners, mutual exchanges should be considered. Many global health programs in highly resourced settings focus exclusively on residents' travel to other countries and do little to host visiting trainees. True exchange programs generally work best within a collaborative context and so should have a mechanism for true exchange. Although visiting residents or doctors from less developed countries may be restricted in offering patient care, they still have open to them many beneficial opportunities for education, observation, and participation in activities. Some examples are described in Chapter 4. One obvious issue is funding; however, anytime funds are procured for residents to go abroad to a "partner" site, those funds might also be used to bring that site's residents or faculty in the other direction. Although some might argue that the money to pay for resident travel helps partner sites, there are counter-arguments. Short trips often accomplish little for host countries unless they are part of a longitudinal, well-planned, and properly supervised program. Visiting residents may worsen "brain drain" in a resource-poor country's institutions by taking up skilled personnel's time for orientation and teaching. Any program visited by international residents or faculty is keenly aware of the resources and time it takes to host visiting scholars. Mutually beneficial exchange programs are challenging to develop and sustain, and usually costly, but creating equal exchange is both an ethical imperative and critical to helping improve global health education through reciprocal experiences for resource-scarce country partners.

One program of note is the Trans-University Centre for Global Health at the University of Virginia. They have developed a true global health exchange program whose benefits can be clearly quantified by the number of students and fellows that continue to produce research papers, community health programs and provide education in global health. Since 1978, this program has trained 80 fellows from 10 countries, all of whom returned to their home countries and have prolific research and teaching careers that promote the health of their communities.[9] Other examples of exchange programs can be found in Chapter 7.

Mentoring

Mentorship is an essential part of all resident training and is no less important for those interested in global health. Residency programs can facilitate mentoring relationships by identifying and supporting faculty members who participate in global health work or have substantial experience in developing countries. A global health mentor for a particular resident can come from a variety of backgrounds and does not necessarily need to be limited to one department (medicine or pediatrics, for examples), as residents can benefit from cross-disciplinary interactions and can thus determine the best fit for their mentor, based on topics or locations of mutual interest. Valuable mentors can also be found in resource-scarce countries that residents visit during international electives. Mentorship agreements should be in writing and meeting times set to review progress.[5]

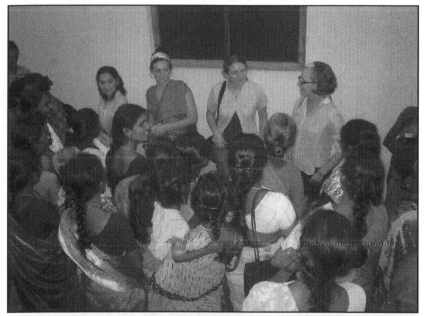

A conversation between students from the Medical School for International Health in Beer Sheva, Israel and students at the Comprehensive Rural Health Project in Jamkhed, Maharashtra, India. (Photo credit: Jonathan Mendelsohn.)

Research

Residents can also learn about global health through collaborative research with institutions in developing countries. Residents may work with investigators conducting research overseas, giving them the chance to learn about basic science and clinical research methods, specific global health topics, and research ethics. Time is often a limiting factor for residents: if a resident intends to do research, expectations must be reasonable to allow for a successful outcome. More often than not, it is easier for a resident to do part of an established project themselves, under the supervision of a faculty research mentor. Those who work in international research know well that projects often move more slowly than anticipated. Institutional Review Board or the Committee on Human Research approval at international sites can take months, even years. Research ethics must be considered: who benefits from research, what is done with the results, and authorship of publications all become important issues in international collaboration. Ideally, these issues are addressed in advance to avoid misunderstandings and resentment as projects move forward. Further discussion of international research can be found in Chapters 3 and 5.

The University of Virginia Center for Global Health Scholars Program creates a competitive research scholarship that assists students in carrying out global health research. This successful program allows students to guide the direction of the research, but also assists students along the way. Each student establishes a steering committee for their project which includes both local and international partners. This committee provides valuable mentorship and guidance through the research cycle.[9] Such established research competitions with specific criteria address challenges that research can pose.

Domestic Educational Experiences in Global Health

Over the last decade, international health has evolved into "global health" as a result of increased globalization and also from the recognition of shared determinants of health in communities throughout the world. Although the global health movement focuses on low- and middle-income countries in an international setting, an overarching goal is to improve the health of underserved and underprivileged people no matter where they live. Local populations in highly-resourced countries also struggle with issues of access and health disparity, providing residency programs with nearby opportunities to expose resident physicians to global health concerns. Opportunities abound in homeless shelters, refugee or immigrant health clinics, travel clinics, and tuberculosis and HIV clinics, in addition to many other sites. Visits to patients living in rooming houses or subsidized housing can be powerful experiences in resource-scarcity. Collaboration with immigrant advocacy groups, legal assistance programs, and similar agencies can help residents acquire skills in working with diverse communities, leadership, activism, and awareness of issues in communities and neighborhoods. Both at home and abroad, language and cultural concordance is a key issue. Access to language and culturally competent care is often limited, and gaining skills in cultural brokerage and use of interpreters is paramount in global health work.

One example is the partnership between the UBC Division of International Health, the Vancouver Native Health Society and Three Bridges Inner City clinic. Both the Vancouver Native Health Society and the Three Bridges clinic provide care to marginalized and special populations in Vancouver (i.e. Immigrant health and gay-lesbian-transsexual health). This collaboration provides a valuable local education for residents to learn skills to apply globally.[7]

Global Health Conferences

Residents should be encouraged to attend and present their research, experiences, and projects at international and national global health conferences. These meetings usually offer excellent didactic teaching and a variety of networking and career opportunities. Examples of such conferences are found in Chapter 8. Most recently the *Global Health Education Consortium* offered Global health career development series in conjunction with their annual conference. This series offered discussion and lecture for medical students and residents on topics from resume preparation to evaluation of field training opportunities. Trainees who attend conferences may solidify their experience by presentation of their experience upon returning to home institutions.

Other Learning Experiences

Experiential learning can also be gained through simulation exercises, such as weekend or overnight experiences that mimic responses to complex humanitarian emergencies. Such experiences teach team building and leadership skills among trainees. Examples of such simulations include 'rich man/poor man' dinners and cultural competency exercises. Experiential exercises are also implemented by organizations such as Doctors Without Borders in training their field staff.

Complementary Degree Programs and Fellowships

Many residents enter medical training after obtaining additional professional degrees or with an interest in pursuing future studies. Global health scholars often pursue a Master's in Public Health (MPH), but other important areas of focus include economics, public policy, international relations and business administration. Some graduate institutions offer degree programs with a focus on global health or have an area of concentration dedicated to it. Master's and doctoral degrees in global health are offered at some institutions. These complementary degree programs provide residents with knowledge and skills beyond clinical medicine. As noted above, some medical schools are beginning to offer residency tracks with an extra year, providing an MPH/residency combination, as well as substantial time abroad to work on projects or research. Examples of these can be found in Chapter 4.

Fellowships in global health are becoming more available, although funding is often a barrier. Many traditional specialty fellowships offer international opportunities. More recently, specific global health fellowships have grown in number. Longer term collaborations are preferable to short rotations, as they offer a greater chance for true collaboration, equal exchange of resources and benefit for the partner institutions and host communities.

Residents often ask about the potential costs and benefits of additional academic training in global health, e.g., earning an MPH degree. Are such degrees helpful? The answer is: "It depends." It depends on the career the resident wants to pursue. For health care professionals engaged in short-term global health assignments or working primarily as clinicians, a public health degree adds little and costs a year of time and money. However, a public health degree can be valuable for professionals in long-term global health assignments and in a wide variety of jobs from field research and overseas training, to program development, implementation, and evaluation. Within MPH studies, specific fields of concentration may have some bearing on a trainee's skill set, but not as important as the mere possession of a public health degree. An MPH provides basic training in epidemiology, bio-statistics, program planning and management, along with one or more content areas such as maternal and child health, health education, and environmental health.

In planning an educational track with complementary degrees and further certification, residents need to know about availability and location of programs, available funding, balance between degree requirements and those of the resident education program, and the potential benefit to the residents' career development. Answering these basic questions may illuminate the need for complementary degrees and certificates.

On a more general note, a variety of questions come up: How does global health relate to public health? Are epidemiology and biostatistics part of the global health core skill set? Is global health just public health in new clothes? What degree of political understanding, economic training, ethics, etc. is needed to prepare those who wish to pursue careers in global health? These are challenging questions for those in medical education trying to develop a global health curriculum. Some answers can be seen in the examples featured in Chapter 4.

Summary

As this chapter has shown, residents have many avenues open to them in pursuing global health education. Global Health is a field that requires didactic instruction and personal study, and clinical field training to solidify learned concepts. There is evidence which suggests that stand-alone international electives are more instructive when presented within a comprehensive global health curriculum.[4] The best programs include a multi-faceted educational approach that includes many, if not all, of the types of programs mentioned in this chapter. The following chapters detail successful program models, considerations on initiating a global health training program, and resources for global health curriculum.

References

[1] Drain PK, Holmes KK, Skeff KM, Hall TL, Gardner P. Global Health Training and International Clinical Rotations During Residency: Current Status, Needs, and Opportunities. Acad Med. 2009 Mar; 84(3):320-325.

[2] Houpt ER, Pearson RD, Hall TL. Three Domains of Competency in Global Health Education: Recommendations for All Medical Students. Acad Med. 2007 Mar; 82 (3):222–225.

[3] Izadnegahdar R, Correia S, Ohata B, Kittler A, ter Kuile S, Vaillancourt S, Saba N, Brewer TF. Global Health in Canadian Medical Education: Current Practices and Opportunities. Acad Med. 2008 Feb; 83 (2): 192-198.

[4] Drain PK, Primack A, Hunt DD, Fawzi WW, Holmes KK, Gardner P. Global Health in Medical Education: A Call for More Training and Opportunities. Acad Med. 2007 Mar; 82 (3):226–230.

[5] Saba N, Brewer TF. Beyond borders: building global health programs at McGill University Faculty of Medicine. Acad Med. 2008 Feb;83(2):185-91.

[6] GHEC on-line learning modules, available at http://globalhealthedu.org/modules/Modules/Default.aspx

[7] University of British Columbia course on Enhanced Skills in Global Health, information available at http://www.familymed.ubc.ca/intl/Education/r3enhancedskills.htm

[8] University of Arizona introduction to global health, information available at http://www.globalhealth.arizona.edu/IHIndex.htm.

[9] Lorntz B, Boissevain JR, Dillingham R, Kelly J, Ballard A, W. Scheld M, Guerrant RL. A Trans-University Center for Global Health. Acad Med. 2008; 83:165–172.

*David Barnard, Thuy Bui, Jack Chase, Evaleen Jones, Scott Loeliger,
Anvar Velji, and Mary T. White*

Introduction

This chapter offers an introduction to the complex ethical issues that arise when training physicians from Western, industrialized countries work overseas in communities with very different cultures, resources, and clinical practices. The first section offers an overview of the historic role of ethics in the medical profession and global health. Following is a discussion of the root of ethical tension and role of conflicting commitments. The third section develops approaches for program assessment, examining the extent to which global health placements meet the training requirements of program directors, the expectations of host supervisors, and satisfy ethical criteria for effective global partnerships. The chapter concludes with case studies and related discussions of practical ethical dilemmas.

An Historical Perspective of Medical Ethics

Primum non nocere ~ First, Do No Harm

For physicians, this hallowed expression of hope and humility, offers recognition that human acts with good intentions may have unwanted consequences. First articulated by Hippocrates and repeated in subsequent medical oaths, it remains the mantra that guides medical decision-making from an ethical point of view. While medical ethicists and journals such as the Hastings Center Report[1] have been considering the ethical implications of modern science and medicine for decades, comparatively little has been written about the ethical implications of medical trainees working abroad. Diverse activities, such as volunteering as a clinician at a hospital in Tanzania, performing obstetrical deliveries in an underserved community in rural Nicaragua, providing HIV care within a PEPFAR-funded center in South Africa, weighing infants in a feeding center in Southeast Asia, or simply attending a community meeting organized by urban community health workers, will require consideration of a resident's effect on individuals, communities and health systems.

Several historical documents central to the ethos of medicine provide important guiding principles. Globally active physicians and trainees should review these documents to gain a deeper, more personal understanding of how ethical concepts are relevant to international practice. The following citations create the necessary framework for promoting change in the global community:

The Physician's Oath (Geneva, September 1948)
The Universal Declaration of Human Rights (Geneva, December 1948)
The European Convention on Human Rights, (Rome, November, 1950)
The Declaration of Alma-Ata; Report of the International Conference on Primary Health
Care (Alma-Ata, September, 1978)

Perhaps the document most relevant to global health is the *Declaration of Alma-Ata,* which established a conceptual basis for the improving the health of the world's nations. The Declaration:

> *strongly reaffirms that health, which is a state of complete physical, mental and social wellbeing, and not merely the absence of disease and infirmity, is a fundamental human right and that the attainment of the highest possible level of health is a most important world-wide social goal whose realization requires the action of many other social and economic sectors in addition to the health sector.*[2]

Citing the inequity of the current state of health care among the World's nations, the meeting of the World Health Organization at Alma-Ata mapped improvements for global health. It emphasized the primacy of collaboration between allied health professionals and the community, accessibility of primary and preventative health care services, use of evidence-based practice, contributions of government and infrastructural development toward health promotion, and the necessity for international collaboration in the effort toward improving wellness of all individuals. These are fundamental concepts necessary for the foundation of global health education among training physicians.

Global Health Ethics for Resident Physicians in Overseas Placements

Residents seek overseas placements for a variety of reasons: to gain clinical experience that is not available at home, to serve patients whose access to health care may otherwise be limited or non-existent, to expand their cultural competency, to contribute positively to under-resourced environments, to conduct research, and to satisfy training requirements at home institutions. Residents may encounter a broad range of ethical issues in these placements due to conflicts within and between four competing ethical commitments: professionalism, service, support, and sustainability. Each of these commitments is critical to the success of residents' overseas experience, and encompasses a number of potential challenges.

Global Health Programs and Partnerships: Four Ethical Commitments

Ethics refers to the moral principles, theories, and conceptual frameworks we use to guide our actions and choices. The variety of ethical approaches commonly used in western medicine may, with some variation in practice, be effectively brought to bear on health care in under-resourced settings. These approaches include the principle of respect for persons, beneficence, non-malfeasance, and justice; consequentialist (ends-based) and deontological (duty-based) theories, virtue ethics, religious ethics, feminist and narrative ethics, and pragmatism. What is new for residents in overseas placements is the diversity of ethical issues that can arise due to unfamiliar environments, cultural norms, environmental stresses and disease demographics, limited resources and infrastructure, and differences in professional expectations.

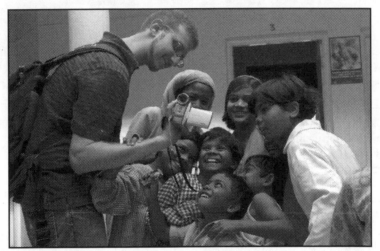

Jonathan Mendelsohn of the Medical School for International Health shows a video to children at an orphanage in a village outside Pune, Maharasthra, India. (Photo credit: Ryan Davis)

Recognition of Ethical Tensions

The primary challenges for rotating residents are to be alert when ethical issues arise and to be willing to pursue the root of ethical tension. Until a conflict is recognized, it cannot be dealt with. As placements are usually in unfamiliar communities and cultures, residents should not expect to be able to recognize or appropriately interpret ethical conflicts until they have spent some time in the host environment. Once residents have begun to understand nuances of local culture, they may find ethical problems everywhere they turn, stemming from differences in assumptions of what constitutes sound clinical practice, professionalism, or even basic judgment.

In grappling with what can often feel frustrating, residents may find it helpful to examine their own expectations and consider why their expectations are not shared in the host community. This kind of awareness calls for keen observation, appreciation of one's own cultural and personal values, and enough knowledge of the host culture and health care environment to have a general idea of where and why differences in values may arise.

Substantial knowledge of the history, culture, environmental, socioeconomic, and political dynamics in the host country and local health systems are extremely helpful in recognizing and effectively negotiating ethical conflicts. It is equally as important to have clear expectations of what is to be accomplished during the rotation—the learning objectives required by the training program at the home institution, the resident's personal goals, and the expectations of the host institution or program. When these are well understood by both the resident and the host country personnel, certain types of ethical conflicts may be minimized.

Ethical issues may arise for residents in their relations with patients, their colleagues, and their host communities. Typically, those involving patients are in the context of clinical care -- the service component of resident placements. Relations with colleagues generally have to do with residents' needs as learners, their responsibilities supporting clinical staff, and potential opportunities for collaboration with their hosts. Ethical issues with the host institution or community as a whole typically have to do with the relationship between the resident's home institution and the overseas host partner and the extent to which this relationship strengthens or burdens the host community over time. Underlying all these relationships are the basic expectations of medical professionals, the details of which vary from place to place with differences in environment, culture, resources, and infrastructure.

The diverse relationships between residents and their patients, colleagues, and host communities, combined with cultural differences and economic disparities between industrialized and developing countries, suggest four ethical commitments in global health placements: *professionalism, service, support, and sustainability.* Ethical issues may arise within each of these commitments, when two or more of these commitments are in conflict, or because a situation that appears to promote some of these values in the short term may over time detract from the same values.

When faced with what appears to be an ethically troubling situation, the first step is always to clarify what is going on. Conflicts of values are usually at the root of most ethical tension; identifying and articulating what those values are often provides a degree of control over the situation. Resolving the conflict then requires determining which values take priority in the situation at hand and what can be done to uphold them. These questions call for judgment, which in turn relies on insight into how the situation is perceived by the involved parties, awareness of one's own values, motivations, and emotional responses, and knowledge of possible alternatives given the particular cultural and institutional contexts.

The following sections explore each of the four commitments: professionalism, service, support, and sustainability, identifying a range of circumstances in each arena that are known to lead to moral distress or ethical conflicts for residents.

Professionalism

The Physician Charter on Professionalism identifies three principles considered fundamental to medical professionalism worldwide: the primacy of patient welfare, respect for patient autonomy, and a commitment to social justice.[3] Each of these is challenged in global health: the first, by the inevitable confusion that arises when physicians' commitments to patient care are impeded by a lack of resources and infrastructure; the second, by the differences in cultural norms, education, and social standing between patients and physicians, and the third by the difficulty of knowing how to engage meaningfully with the elusive goal of social justice. The Charter also identifies a number of expectations fundamental to medical professionalism:

- clinical competence and life-long learning
- honesty with patients
- ensuring informed consent and error management
- confidentiality
- maintaining appropriate relations with patients
- improving access to care
- "wise and effective management" of health care resources
- duties to uphold and promote advances in medical knowledge
- managing conflicts of interest appropriately
- effective collaboration with other professionals in the interests of patient care
- establishing and monitoring standards for professional training
- remediating, disciplining, and censoring those who fail to meet those standards

Of these, the expectations that only involve the resident, such as clinical competence and maintaining appropriate relations with patients, are straightforward. But in non-Western, less-developed countries, most of these professional expectations will be upheld in ways that differ, sometimes considerably, from what residents are used to. Residents will want to remind themselves daily that their professional expectations may differ from those of their host colleagues. This awareness will facilitate effective management of ethical conflicts and is probably the resident's best defense against frustration.

Tourism and recreation: Most residents drawn to overseas rotations love the adventure of travel, new environments, and new experiences. But among the many medical professionals who work overseas, there are those who have use their placements primarily as a "medical safari," or base camp for recreational tourism. Residents will be watched by their hosts, and if repeatedly absent, may be perceived as using their overseas placements to take a vacation. While some recreational exploration is understandable, as representatives of their countries, profession, and home institutions, residents are responsible not only for themselves but for the future of their program or partnership, and should conduct themselves with that in mind.

Licensing, service, and accountability: Again, as visitors, residents will often need to obtain a medical license in order to take primary responsibility for patient care. If a license is not obtained, they may still contribute to patient care but their clinical activities will be overseen by a supervising physician. That said, for a variety of reasons, it is not uncommon for host country supervisors to be absent at times, leaving the resident in charge of patient care. This can place residents in an ethical bind: whether to do their best to meet patient needs without adequate licensing or oversight, or to withhold necessary care that may be urgent and that they think they are capable of providing. This is a common ethical conflict in which professionalism—the duty not to practice without a license or to exceed the bounds of one's training—runs up against the commitment to service, where the resident may well be able to provide competent care, absent which patients will suffer. In such circumstances, residents will rely on their best judgment to find the solution that fits the circumstances, drawing on their perceptions of patient need, their clinical abilities, potential consequences for themselves, their patients, their supervisors, their programs, and available alternatives. What is never conscionable is for residents to use such opportunities to "practice" their clinical skills. Unfortunately, this form of opportunism does happen, invariably tarnishing relations between visitors and their hosts.

Service

The goals for residents in overseas placements typically include gaining experience with unfamiliar disease patterns in environments with scarce resources, strengthening the local health care system through patient care and teaching, and perhaps undertaking research projects. A few common ethical concerns that may arise in the course of clinical service include the following:

Residents as learners: Residents are attracted to overseas placements for the rich learning opportunities they provide. For their first few weeks, residents will learn how to work with limited resources, treating conditions they have never seen before, in an unknown environment, sometimes where they do not speak the local language. As learners, they can burden their hosts until they become acquainted with their new environment, practice patterns, and support staff. For this reason, the first responsibility of the resident is to come as prepared as possible and to commit to rapidly becoming a productive member of the medical staff. Inevitably, residents will be exposed to circumstances and practices that take getting used to. Common frustrations include a lack of functioning medical equipment, scarcity of basic supplies and pharmaceuticals, and fluctuating water and power supplies. How residents manage the adjustment may occasionally merit psychological attention or ethical concern, but simply being aware that adjustment can be challenging may alleviate stress.

Clinical Practice: In settings with limited resources, clinical practice differs in numerous ways from that of industrialized countries. Physicians and patients may have very different notions of what constitutes health or disease, what is expected to happen when seen by a doctor, and how they understand disease causation and medical treatment. In less-developed countries, diagnoses will usually rely more on clinical skills than laboratory test results, and treatments may involve non-specific use of fluctuating supplies of limited medications. For physicians used to accurate diagnoses and targeted interventions, some clinical approaches may at first seem strange, inefficient, inappropriate, or incorrect. As at home, residents will want to keep in mind that their host physicians have knowledge and experience that they lack, and question practices judiciously with the expectation that much of what they question can reasonably be explained. Once past the novelty, learning how to diagnose and treat patients with limited resources is one of the most important skill sets that residents can bring home.

Record-keeping: In industrialized health systems, medical records serve a variety of purposes: as a document of patient care, legal evidence, research data, and billing record. But where paper and pencils are in short supply, record keeping may be very limited. Adapting to clinical settings where detailed record keeping is not the norm is one more challenge residents should be prepared to encounter. Such challenges are not without recourse, and in the case of medical records, for example, residents may be able to share knowledge and practice from their home institution in order to begin collaborative discussion, possibly helping to analyze and improve clinical practice in the host community. It is critical to approach all such discussions with a spirit of equality, as both the host and visitor have valuable knowledge and experience to contribute

Long-range planning: In health systems in industrialized countries, monitoring resources, keeping plentiful supplies, maintaining equipment, and overseeing usage patterns are routine. Where resources are abundant, it is common to anticipate the future, to plan ahead, and to take action to minimize risk. But in many developing countries this kind of planning ahead is often not possible. As a result, the focus defaults to the present. In clinics and hospitals, the focus on the present may result in failure to maintain equipment, disruptions in basic supplies, long waits to see a physician or to get supplies, and little regard for notions of conservation or triage. For patients, the inability to plan ahead or control uncertainty are often met with a sense of inevitability and fatalism; the family is where one turns for material support, and the efficacy of healing is often attributed to God or Providence. These differing attitudes toward uncertainty, time, resource use, and human agency will vary with individuals, cultures, and circumstances, but they are worth noticing in any setting as they will govern much of day to day operations.

Paternalism, Autonomy and Informed Consent: Whereas in highly-resourced, westernized medical culture the doctor-patient relationship is characterized by patient autonomy, other countries the physician-patient relationship is characterized more by paternalism. There are a number of reasons for this, some having to do with differences in education, gender, and social class. Whatever the reason, many patients will not expect to be involved in medical decisions or to have their preferences solicited and respected; instead, they will expect physicians to be the experts and will do as they are instructed by their medical provider. For these patients, being asked to participate in decisions may even be unsettling. But as in all cultures, physician-patient dynamics will vary with individuals. Some host-country physicians do make an effort to involve patients in decisions, and some patients ask many questions.

Truth-telling: Just as expectations regarding informed consent can vary with individual physicians and patients, what patients and families are told about diagnoses and prognoses, especially when conditions are serious or terminal, may also vary between individuals and cultures. In some cultures, depending on the diagnosis, patients will not expect or want to be informed—being told the truth may be considered a violation of their rights or as destroying the possibility for hope. Other may want to know.

Residents will want to watch their host colleagues carefully when caring for patients with terminal illnesses and become familiar with local practice patterns in end-of-life care.

Importantly, in some settings, patients may be accompanied by family members who are responsible for providing food, washing clothes and bedding, and dispensing medications. This "carer" or family member may be the person with whom the physician interacts the most. Being aware of who is providing supportive care for patients can therefore be important, sometimes raising ethical issues, especially if the carer is a young child or otherwise of questionable ability to understand what is needed. (Note: where having a carer is essential, someone must usually leave school or the workplace which can create other kinds of hardships for a family, sometimes lapses in care, and incentives for the patient to return home as quickly as possible.)

Confidentiality: In open wards, privacy and confidentiality may be difficult to sustain, even when physicians speak very softly. Despite lack of privacy, confidentiality is of critical importance, especially with conditions that may carry stigma such as cancer or HIV. As a widely-prevalent case example, HIV raises complex ethical problems. In some parts of the world, men may resist testing as a positive diagnosis suggests weakness. Women may seek testing more often than men, but in countries where women have few rights, being diagnosed with HIV may result in abuse or being forced out of the home. As with any sexually transmitted disease, residents should be aware that partner notification may not be expected or may need to be handled very carefully. Confidentiality is an area where assumptions are best avoided and local norms learned quickly.

Gender raises a host of ethical issues that vary across cultures. In many cultures, while women may have important social roles that carry considerable respect, their legal rights are limited. While women provide support for their partners, raise children, and contribute to family income, and they may lack rights to property, control over money they have earned, and a voice in their own health care decisions. For a geographically isolated woman, the cost of transportation to a clinic or regional hospital may be more than she or her spouse can afford to spend. When seen by a physician, her partner may expect to be present and may wish to speak for her—indeed, this may be what she expects as well. Visiting residents will want to learn about local gender norms and expectations and find ways of adapting that will permit necessary information exchange. Especially troubling are domestic violence and abuse where women have few legal rights, limited social standing, and there are few safe alternatives.

Traditional medicine: In many developing countries, patients and their families may have health beliefs that invoke religious or supernatural beliefs, and/or confidence that traditional healers may be necessary and effective. Traditional approaches to health care and healing can be fascinating, revealing much about how individuals understand disease causality, the "sick role," and their moral responsibilities. Traditional healers may make effective use of local plant-based remedies; they may also cause real harm. If a patient has confidence in a particular healer and wishes to make use of traditional medicine, there may be some benefit in making the effort to do so. But when and how to integrate traditional practices into allopathic medicine will probably need to be determined on a case by case basis. Residents would again be advised to watch their host colleagues handle such requests. The default position should be to go with the best clinical practices possible under the circumstances. Treatment aside, learning as much as possible about traditional medicine and health beliefs can strengthen residents' cultural knowledge and relationships with patients and colleagues, and in some cases, may be valuable clinical information.

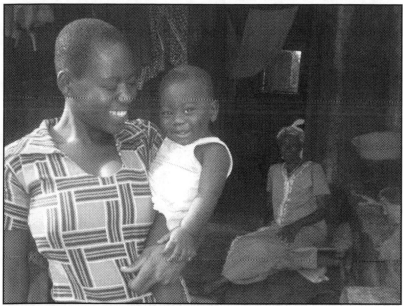

A qualitative project interviewing women in northern Ghana about their use of contraceptives. Sponsored by the Bixby Center for Population, Health, and Sustainability at UC Berkeley. (Photo credit: Sirina Keesara.)

Support

Residents are invited to developing countries in part for the opportunities they offer to their host colleagues and local health systems. All residents potentially provide knowledge, skills, resources, and collaboration opportunities, but if and how these are realized will be up to individuals. Residents will want to think about how to most effectively engage with the needs of their host colleagues and host institution. Some opportunities and potential hazards are described below.

Medical errors: Self-regulation is a central element of medical professionalism that requires physicians to monitor errors and near misses with the expectation of correction and ongoing pursuit of excellence. But if and how personal criticism is given and taken varies enormously across cultures. Ideally, residents should talk with their hosts in advance about what to do when they make medical mistakes and what to tell patients and colleagues. Similarly, how residents should respond if they witness a host colleague mishandle a patient or make a major mistake will likely vary from what is done at home. Self-regulation is always sensitive; it is all the more so when visiting physicians are involved.

Teaching: Residents bring a great deal of knowledge with them and may be asked to teach their host colleagues or medical students. This is one way residents can positively support their colleagues and medical community and strengthen the institutional partnership. But before launching into any teaching, it is usually helpful to ask enough questions to get a sense of what the audience already knows, and as best as is possible, to tailor one's teaching to what is possible in the host medical community.

Research: Another important need to which residents can contribute is research and publication. The 90/10 global health disparity -- that 90% of the world's disease burden, primarily responsible for illness in under-resourced nations and communities, is supported by only 10% of the world's research funding -- reflects the need for increased research and publication on health care in developing countries. Some of this research is already happening, but is usually designed and conducted by westerners. One of the greatest needs in global health is for indigenous researchers in developing countries to learn to design, conduct, and publish their work in journals that are publicly available. Building research capacity in these countries is a huge task, requiring funding, trained personnel, research oversight, regional or national journals devoted to global health and access to published literature. Ethical issues involved in human subject research are complex and variable, well exceeding the scope of this chapter, encompassing vulnerable populations, informed consent, benefit sharing, diverse forms of exploitation, use of placebo controls, and more. Nonetheless, even without engaging in major clinical studies, residents on short-term placements may support local research initiatives. Because research training tends to be limited in developing countries, residents may contribute by teaching their colleagues how to conduct a needs assessment, a literature search, develop a research question, find funding, and write grants. If they anticipate returning, they may invite host colleagues to collaborate on a research project of their own. Each of those activities provides tangible support for individuals, and indirectly, strengthens host country health systems and institutions.

Publication: Writing for publication may also be challenging for medical professionals in developing countries. In the absence of ready access to journals or the internet, strong language and writing skills, and knowledge of the publication process, many fine researchers in developing countries have difficulty getting their work published and disseminated. Residents with experience in research or writing can provide valuable support by offering grant-writing or editing assistance and helping host-country colleagues find appropriate journals and on-line publishing opportunities for their work. These activities can in turn advance individual careers, contribute to global health care knowledge, and ultimately strengthen health care capacities worldwide.

Brain drain: Research conducted in developing countries may provide a number of short-term benefits that are attractive to host institutions: jobs, infrastructure, drugs, supplies, computers and other technology, training, publication opportunities, and more. But in the process, researchers often draw on local health care staff to facilitate their research, generally people who are fluent in the local language who can effectively communicate with research participants. When external salaries or other opportunities are compelling, indigenous staff will be easily drawn away from their usual clinical duties. This siphoning off of skilled health workers from the institutions and patients that rely on them has the effect of an internal brain drain. In parts of the world where research or development projects are abundant, this brain drain can be considerable. Similarly, by bringing in quantities of free medical supplies and drugs, researchers can disrupt local pharmacies and businesses. In these and other ways, short-term global health projects can impose hidden costs on local communities. International partnerships, even those undertaken with the goal of strengthening local community health care capacities, must therefore be carefully designed in anticipation of their foreseeable and unforeseeable consequences.

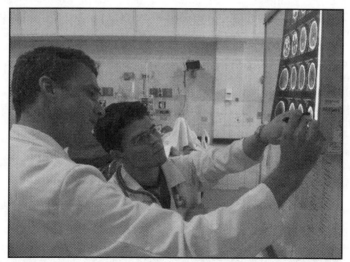

Dr. Robert Fuller, attending physician in emergency medicine from the University of Connecticut, reviews a patient's CT scan with David Aragundi, an Ecuadorian medical student, at Hospital Luis Vernaza in Guayaquil, Ecuador. (Photographer: Benjamin Silverberg.)

Sustainability

The Physician's Charter identifies the commitment to social justice as one of the guiding principles of medical professionalism. What constitutes "social justice" is not specified. In the context of global health, Western physicians often use this term to promote international aid programs, whether of humanitarian disaster relief or development. But while our discomfort with the vast economic disparities between nations prompts calls for social justice, what can or should be done to rectify disparities remains politically and practically elusive. Critiques of global aid efforts have been mounting in recent years, pointing out that despite a trillion dollars worth of monetary aid to the African continent since the 1960s, most African countries are experiencing greater poverty, health care need, and political tension than they were forty years ago.[4] There are numerous reasons given for this, most notably political interests behind the aid industry which have long permitted corrupt governments to prosper. Other factors include the population explosion across the continent since 1960 which creates serious social, economic, medical, and environmental stressors, "learned helplessness" fostered by habituated reliance on external aid to solve local problems, and top-down, theory-driven aid efforts that have not included host country perspectives or personnel in leadership positions and are rarely assessed or held accountable for outcomes.

So what should be done? What *can* be done? Regardless of the difficulties of providing aid effectively, it is now clear that international security calls for effective and lasting public health and health care systems in every corner of the globe. The increasing incidence of infectious disease which can travel the world in a few days calls for rigorous monitoring of disease outbreaks everywhere. This kind of surveillance requires vigilance in local clinics by trained health care personnel, record-keeping capabilities, communication systems, containment capacities, and more. A question of some urgency today is how industrialized nations, which have long benefitted from the best and the brightest medical graduates from developing countries, can now contribute to the development of strong, indigenous, sustainable, health care systems everywhere in the world.

This question needs to be at the forefront of international partnerships and residency placements. While the ultimate goal--effective health systems worldwide--calls for investment and leadership well beyond the reach of any individual or program, visiting physicians, residents, researchers, and others involved in global health partnerships can nonetheless consider that their overseas placements may offer leadership examples and other meaningful opportunities to their host colleagues. Medical residents are in effect ambassadors of their native countries, cultures, and profession. Demonstrating quality patient care, collegiality, initiative, accountability, eagerness to learn and a willingness to share what they know, can communicate volumes and sometimes inspire new ways of thinking. A risk for residents and other visitors is that because of their skills and motivation, they may be encouraged to take on major responsibilities and leadership roles. But they must hold back, aware that the growth and sustainability of effective health systems relies on developing indigenous leadership.

The goals of sustainable health systems can only be achieved through carefully designed and coordinated training programs, mentoring, and infrastructure development. Each of these is clearly beyond the reach of visiting medical residents. What they can do is to become familiar with the cultures, needs, and people on the ground. By working closely with professionals and lay people, medical residents will have knowledge that development planners often lack. Sharing this knowledge when they return home is an unquestionably vital role that residents can play in contributing to goals of social justice.

This section has been a short introduction to the broad range of social and ethical issues western medical residents can expect to encounter when working in developing countries. This is just a beginning—it is impossible to comprehensively capture the variety and complexity of ethical conflicts that can arise between people and communities with vastly different cultures, languages, and resources. Our hope is that being aware of where conflicts of ethical and professional values can arise will help to make transitions easier, conflicts manageable, and global health experiences more rewarding for residents and their hosts. But while they go abroad to learn, residents return with additional responsibilities. In the effort to strengthen health systems around the world, they are important resources and we need to hear from them. Their final ethical responsibility is to come home and to share what they have learned.

Assessing the Ethics of Global Health Training Experiences

Before carrying out an ethical assessment of a global health training program, the evaluator has several choices to make: (1) what aspects of the program should be evaluated? (2) according to what norms will the evaluation be conducted? (3) what indicators will be relied upon to demonstrate whether and to what extent the norms are being met? Crump and Sugarman, for example, have suggested four ethically significant stakeholders whose interests could be the focus of a comprehensive assessment: (1) patients and other intended beneficiaries, (2) trainees, (3) local staff and host institutions, and (4) sending institutions.[5] As an overarching governing norm they propose "mutual and reciprocal benefit" for all stakeholders, the optimistic corollary to the precept *primum non nocere* with which this chapter began. In common with most commentators, however, Crump and Sugarman omit any discussion of specific indicators that could help a program director determine the extent to which his or her program is approximating its chosen norm with respect to any of its stakeholders.

In this section we will outline an approach to program evaluation, expressed in the form of three questions.

1. How well does the program help the residents anticipate and prepare for the ethical challenges they are likely to meet in their international placements?
2. How conscientiously do the residents attempt to fulfill their professional ethical obligations in their placements?
3. What is the impact on the host community of accommodating the educational objectives of the program?

We will accept as our overarching norm the obligation to pursue the greatest possible net balance of benefit over harm, with respect both to our trainees and to host communities. (We are mindful that in emphasizing this consequentialist formulation of our governing norm we seem to be leaving out of account some other significant elements of ethical evaluation that are independent of consequences, e.g., whether actions conform to a moral rule, respect rights, or express a moral virtue. We will have occasion to refer to these important perspectives below.) We will then briefly suggest some indicators that might be helpful in determining the extent to which we have achieved this goal.

How well does the program help the residents anticipate and prepare for the ethical challenges they are likely to meet in their international placements?

We noted above that residents' ability to function conscientiously and respectfully in their international setting requires them to possess substantial knowledge of local history, culture, environment, and contemporary political dynamics, as well as the socioeconomic conditions of the local population, and the nature of the local health system. To this we might add the impact of the global economic and political system on the ability of the national government to make and carry out policies for health and social welfare. Accordingly, some basic preparatory work should be required of residents prior to their departure. Some useful indicators of a program's ability to provide this preparation would include:

- Content experts in relevant disciplines and area studies participate in residents' didactic curriculum, including representatives from the local communities where possible.
- Residents learn research methods for gathering relevant country- and community-level information on, e.g., social determinants of health; health indicators disaggregated according to gender, ethnicity, socioeconomic status, and geography; status of the enjoyment or violation of internationally recognized human rights;

local resources for health and human rights advocacy; global macroeconomic context for national policy making.

- Residents anticipate and analyze paradigm cases of ethical conflict (similar to those in the previous section) through oral discussion and written analysis.
- Local mentors are selected and remunerated in part for their ability to provide appropriate supervision and feedback for residents' encounters with social and cultural issues, as well as for their clinical abilities.

How conscientiously do the residents attempt to fulfill their professional ethical obligations in their placements?

We observed earlier in this chapter that residents may play several roles during their placements, including, e.g., physician, teacher, learner, colleague, researcher, and guest. Within each of these there are role-specific norms, expectations, and obligations that provide a pattern and context for conscientious professional behavior. While it would greatly exceed the bounds of this section to elaborate in any detail these norms and obligations, about which ethicists can and do sometimes disagree, there is broad agreement on the considerations that ought to be taken into account in determining one's ethical responsibilities in a given situation. Thus, as suggested above, conscientious ethical deliberation should begin by *identifying the stakeholders* affected by one's actions. Then, with respect to those stakeholders, we should attempt to identify the *consequences* (in terms of benefits and harms) of our actions; *duties* that we might have toward affected persons that are independent of particular consequences (such as being truthful, protecting confidentiality, keeping a promise, or respecting a right), and commitments *inherent to the identity of a professional*, such as the priority of patient welfare over personal gain, and the responsibility to maintain and enforce professional standards.

The evaluator's question then becomes the extent to which the resident has internalized the commitment to acting according to these norms, and how well he or she has succeeded in doing so. Data for answering these questions might be collected either contemporaneously or retrospectively, depending on resources and telecommunications capabilities. For example, if residents can be in simultaneous contact during their time abroad by email, telephone, or videoconferencing, they can present current cases or issues that raise ethical concerns and demonstrate their commitment and ability to analyze them according to the terms in the preceding paragraph. Alternatively—and possibly more realistically given constraints of time and resources—residents can provide retrospective written analyses of cases or issues at the conclusion of their rotation, participate in oral debriefing, or both. Useful indicators that the resident had met the expectations for ethically responsible conduct would include:

- The resident identifies a comprehensive, if not exhaustive, range of affected stakeholders.
- The resident identifies relevant, role-specific norms and obligations.
- The resident draws appropriately on knowledge of social, cultural, political conditions in the community.
- The resident reasons logically and coherently in applying the norms, professional obligations, and local knowledge to the case at hand.
- The local mentor confirms (or disconfirms) the resident's self-report via independent observation and feedback to the program director that reflects the local community's value system and priorities.

These indicators are useful complements to evaluation of the resident's "professionalism" as suggested by the ACGME, which uses categories such as: always demonstrates respect, compassion, integrity, honesty; teaches/role models responsible behavior; shows total commitment to self-assessment; willingly acknowledges errors; readily places needs of others above self-interest.[6]

What is the impact on the host community of accommodating the educational objectives of the program?

Of the various possible effects that the program might have on the local community, those that are likely to be of greatest interest are also the least likely to be determinable, namely, the effects on the health of the local population. After all, what could be a more direct measure of host-community benefit or harm than improvements or deterioration in important population health indicators that are attributable to the community's hosting of a residency placement? As with most clinical interventions themselves, however, there are simply too many confounding factors, and the likely effect sizes too small, to permit such a causal connection even if we could agree on which health indicators to use. Nevertheless, if we are to advance beyond merely exhorting programs to produce "mutual and reciprocal benefit," we should try to develop more specific, measurable indicators that can contribute to this assessment.

If the residency placement is to be a genuinely collaborative partnership with the host community, which is itself the first requirement for an ethically sound program, the selection of these indicators of community impact must be a shared process between the sending program and the hosts. Because each community will have its own social and health-related characteristics, and each host institution will have its own priorities and expectations, we cannot specify any particular set of indicators as a general prescription.

We would like to suggest, however, that a promising resource for the partners to use in developing their indicators is the "normative framework for the right to health" developed by the Committee on Economic, Social, and Cultural Rights in its *General Comment 14 on The Right to the Highest Attainable Standard of Health (Article 12 of the International Covenant on Economic, Social, and Cultural Rights)*. The Committee developed its framework as a guide to States Parties to the Covenant on Economic, Social, and Cultural Rights to help them evaluating their compliance with their legal obligations under the Covenant to "respect, protect, and fulfill" the right to health for their inhabitants.

The Committee identified several *health system characteristics* that States Parties—and the treaty bodies and human rights advocates monitoring them—could use to assess treaty compliance:

- Availability (of health services and facilities)
- Physical accessibility
- Economic accessibility (affordability)
- Acceptability (cultural respect, gender and life-cycle sensitivity, respect for confidentiality)
- Quality (skilled personnel, approved and unexpired drugs and equipment, safe and potable water, sanitation)

And the Committee identified *issues and groups* of "special concern":

- Non-discrimination
- Gender perspective
- Children and adolescents
- Older persons
- Persons with disabilities
- Indigenous peoples

These health system characteristics, and the quality of care provided to these populations, could be the basis for a meaningful assessment of what we might call the "ethics and human rights impact" of global health residency placements. The challenge would be to design quantitative measures—for example, clinic waiting times, patients seen per day, births attended by skilled personnel—that could be tracked in settings with and without, before and after, the presence of trainees and whose fluctuations could be plausibly attributed at least in part to the host community's participation in the training program. Even granting the epistemological and methodological difficulties of designing such measures, the very act of paying attention to these aspects of the placements—as a collaborative effort of senders and hosts—is a salutary recognition of the moral dimensions of global health education.

Cases for Discussion

The following cases are focused on residency trainees in global health placements, and provide a framework for discussion using the concepts introduced in this chapter.

Case 1: David is a pediatrics intern on an elective in a large public hospital in Uganda. He is part of a group of students listening to a senior physician on bedside rounds. They are clustered around the bed of a 4-year old boy who likely has acute bacterial meningitis. The patient's mother and sister are present, as the physician discusses the risk of death and disability. The hospital ward is undivided, and other patients, families, and staff are listening. The physician turns to David and asks him to do a lumbar puncture – something he has never done before but would love to learn how to do. David feels concerned about the way that the discussion can be heard throughout the ward, and about how he will obtain consent given that he does not speak the local language. He questions whether he is the most appropriate provider for this procedure, and whether the patient's family will even be able to afford the necessary antibiotics if the diagnosis is confirmed.

This case illustrates a) of the need for preservation of patient privacy and confidentiality b) the challenges to informed consent, c) matching responsibility to ability and d) issues of affordability and limited resources.

a) Patient Privacy-Confidentiality:
Even under ideal circumstances, confidentiality can be difficult to achieve. Bedside rounds allow for a discussion of the patient's case history between medical educators and students. At times, multiple patients may share a room and in some settings, patients are treated in adjacent beds in large wards. Families frequently provide nursing and supportive care to patients in under-resourced settings, and are therefore privy to discussions about other patients. Adding dividing curtains and screens does not entirely mitigate these circumstances, and may not be financially feasible. However, appropriate gowning of patients, draping and other barriers provide partial psychological "security" to patients and families. In the case of this discussion about a child with meningitis, the teaching points of physical diagnosis and the review of potential sequelae (e.g. death, disability) would ideally be conducted in a semi-private space with a culturally concordant interpreter for the family, or alternatively the discussion of prognosis reviewed with family in a separate space and at a separate time from teaching to trainees about the illness.

b) Challenges to Informed Consent:
While widely practiced in settings with western medical ethics, the notion of informed consent in other nations is highly variable, and culturally dependant. While some communities value individual autonomy, in others, consent is obtained through families or via tribal hierarchy. This complexity is compounded by language barriers, variation in levels of education, and differing conceptions of health, wellness and scientific principles. Even the notion of information is dependent on the situation, and some patients may want to avoid any discussion of the medical details of their illness. The process of informed consent may best be performed in tandem, with an interpreter or cultural broker, who can both teach the trainee about the salient linguistic and cultural norms specific to the setting, while conveying the relevant information to the patient or surrogate decision maker in an appropriate level of detail. By aligning with a local interpreter, medical trainees may also accomplish increased "buy in" from the patient or decision-maker, by demonstrating connection to the community and sensitivity to cultural issues specific to the host community. This process should be undertaken and reflected upon with perspective on the visiting trainees own ethical framework.

c) Trainee Professionalism:
Due to the under-resourced staffing in many international placements, as well as to the respect afforded to medical trainees from highly resourced, western training centers, visiting medical trainees may be offered the opportunity to perform medical tasks at a high level of responsibility and complexity. The availability of these opportunities is not a surrogate for judgment about a trainee's qualification for the task. Prior to performing all treatments or procedures, especially those that are new or unfamiliar, trainees should review their level of training, the procedural and biomedical details of the case, and the process of consent with their host supervisors.
 As medical documentation varies between settings, it is also critical to review with host physicians or staff how and if documentation is accomplished. In this reflection process, if a trainee feels under-qualified for the complexity or the risk of a given situation, they must communicate this to the supervising provider – and not allow opportunity to dictate responsibility.

d) Issues of Resource Scarcity:
One of the major barriers in providing healthcare in under-resourced communities is the paucity of supplies or medication. In such situations, it may be of limited benefit to perform invasive tests or procedures on a patient, especially in geographically or economically isolated settings, unless treatments are available in a timely and geographically appropriate manner. The recommendation or performance of diagnostic maneuvers may be understood by a patient or a family as implying that the treatment is

49

readily available depending on the results. Even if a patient may be diagnosed and a treatment is available, the patient or their family may not be able to wait for an entire course of therapy due to economic or safety constraints. For these reasons, trainees should carefully consider the balance of benefit and risk to the patient, as well as to discuss with patients and families, the details of treatment availability, duration, and cost prior to performing invasive diagnostic tests or treatments.

Case 2: Ayana is a second year resident in internal medicine in the United States, interested in pursuing an infectious disease fellowship. She is fluent in Spanish, and has previously participated in volunteer humanitarian and medical trips to rural communities in Central America. She has become particularly interested in Leishmaniasis, and would like to conduct a research project on disease prevalence in rural Northeastern Guatemala. She will take skin biopsies of patients with Leishmaniasis ulcers, and send them to a laboratory for analysis. The population in the planned study community does not have widespread access to medical care, and standard treatments for Leishmaniasis are not available there. The community is very rural, 200 kilometers from the nearest city hospital, and most of the residents are subsistence farmers. The average education completed by the local residents is the fourth grade. Ayana worries that study participants will not understand that the study will likely not result in treatment for them. Although she is hopeful that other residents will continue her work in the following years, Ayana is not sure about the sustainability of the research effort in this region. Finally, she is concerned that the local physician, with whom she has worked in the past, will see her study as exploiting the local population for her gain as a physician from a more highly resourced nation.

This case illustrates a) the challenge of human subject research in communities not familiar with the practice of medical research b) issues of sustainability in resident-driven global health research c) resident-host physician relationships in global health collaboration.

a) Human subject research is a complex and time-consuming process, even in highly resourced medical settings. Many communities in global health settings may not be familiar with the concept of medical research – especially, the idea that research is not usually designed to directly benefit the participants, but instead may provide benefit for future generations. Furthermore, informed consent, a critical part of the research process, may be complicated by linguistic and cultural barriers in unfamiliar study communities. As mentioned in *Case 1*, the concept of informed consent may clash with local concepts of decision-making. Enlisting a local interpreter to serve as a cultural broker may help visiting residents to understand the nuances of the host community. Providing thorough explanation at a level of complexity appropriate for the local community, if possible at a community meeting, or via local public health workers, may help to inform local populations about the purpose of a study and the potential risks and benefits of participation. Consideration of low literacy among both research subjects and project participants may lead to pictorial or verbal demonstrations instead of written explanation. Finally, providing training and supplies as appropriate compensation – such as educating study participants on vector control and donating bed nets in a community affected by insect-borne disease – may sustainably decrease disease burden and increase mutual collaboration for future research, even if the current project does not result in clinical cure for participants.

b) One of the greatest challenges in global health work with underserved communities is continuity of effort once the international volunteers have left the host community. Sustainability and institutional memory can be difficult to accomplish especially with limited budgets, differences in priorities between visiting and host collaborators and geographic or technologic isolation of the host community. Prior to beginning a research or clinical project, long range planning is key, ideally carried out in consultation with senior physicians or researchers with knowledge in both the subject area and in the geographic and cultural specifics of the planned study community. Engaging local experts in the host community (physicians, nurses, public health researchers) early in the planning process, will help to refine study proposals and give insight into prior local research that may not have been widely distributed. Conducting a needs assessment in the host community – if possible involving host community members as well as medical and local government or healthy ministry officials – can increase community engagement and lead to connections with local colleagues who may provide institutional memory as well as a sustainable work force if such funding exists.

c) Fostering successful host physician-volunteer relationships is an integral part of a fulfilling global health experience. In *Case 2*, the perception of an international medical volunteer as profiting from disease in the local community may be damaging to productive collegial interaction. Co-authoring research publications may help to engage local physicians and medical personnel, as well as present opportunities to share research and technological skills among colleagues. Scientific needs assessment with local allied health professionals and health ministry officials may increase host personnel interest and engagement. Finally, developing funding that supports training of previously underemployed local residents, may lead to skill-building for future employment, and combat "brain-drain" by increasing the health workforce.

References

51

[1] The Hastings Center Report can be found at http://www.thehastingscenter.org.
[2] The Declaration of Alma-Ata, http://www.who.int/hpr/NPH/docs/declaration_almaata.pdf, accessed June 16, 2009.
[3] The ABIM Foundation, ACP–ASIM Foundation, and European Federation of Internal Medicine (2002) Medical Professionalism in the New Millennium: A Physician Charter. *Annals of Internal Medicine* 136(3): 243-246.
[4] Moya, D (2009) *Dead aid : why aid is not working and how there is a better way for Africa.* New York : Farrar, Straus and Giroux.
[5] Crump, JA., Sugarman, J. (2008) *Ethical Considerations for Short-term Experiences by Trainees in Global Health.* JAMA, 300: pp1456-1458.
[6] AGCME indicators accessible at www.acgme.org.
-- Gostin, LO (2008) *Global Health - Meeting Basic Survival Needs of the World's Least Healthy People: Toward a Framework Convention on Global Health.* The Georgetown Law Journal, Vol 96 (331).
-- Committee on the US Commitment to Global Health; Institute of Medicine (2009) *The U.S Commitment to Global Health: Recommendations for the Public and Private Sectors.* National Academy of Sciences. Available at: http://www.nap.edu/catlog/12642.html. Accessed June 16, 2009.

*Melanie Anspacher, Thomas Hall, Julie Herlihy, Chi-Cheng Huang,
Suzinne Pak Gorstein, and Nicole St Clair*

Introduction

Residency programs in the United States are undergoing an exciting period of growth focused on global health. The increased interest likely stems from globalization and the greater involvement of medical students, residents, and faculty in global health activities. Currently, many residency programs lack an established consensus on global health competencies and validated evaluation tools for residents, curricula, and residency tracks in global health.

The Accreditation Council for Graduate Medical Education (ACGME) has designed six general competencies which serve as broad domains for directing resident education. These areas are subdivided into more specific goals and objectives. This chapter provides global health curriculum guidelines based on the ACGME competencies and a sample fund-of-knowledge checklist to help ensure that trainees achieve the skills needed for effective international experiences. Suggestions for implementation of a competency-based curriculum in a variety of medical disciplines are given. The chapter concludes with suggestions for evaluating residents and programs based on these competencies.[1]

Competency-Based Guidelines for Residency-Based Global Health Programs

With specific examples for programs in Pediatrics, Obstetrics and Gynecology, Family Medicine and Internal Medicine

In an effort to establish discipline-specific global health curricular standards for resident education, we provide these suggested guidelines for residency global health training. The guidelines were adapted from the competency-based goals and objectives developed by the American Academy of Pediatrics Section on International Child Health (SOICH) working group on Pediatric Resident Education.[2] They are generalized to include all patient populations. Additionally, we include examples of how to tailor the competencies for residency programs in pediatrics, obstetrics and gynecology, and internal medicine; with the understanding that trainees in family medicine would achieve competencies in all three areas of expertise. We chose these fields because they provide the majority of primary care in resource-limited settings.

Please note that these examples are not all-encompassing, but instead are intended to be used as a guideline for global health training programs and adapted according to each medical discipline's needs. For example, surgical residency programs should incorporate procedural-based competencies for their trainees. We encourage each program to incorporate their own objectives, both specific to their field of expertise and to their international study site.

Competency 1: Patient Care
Provide family-centered care that is age-appropriate, compassionate, and effective for the treatment of health problems and the promotion of health.

OBJECTIVES:

1. Demonstrate a logical and **appropriate clinical approach** to the care of patients in a developing country setting, utilizing **local resources** and **international standardized guidelines.**

2. Provide **culturally sensitive care and support** to patients and families.

3. Participate in **health promotion and injury/disease prevention** activities in an international setting, utilizing local guidelines and practices.

4. Describe and practice a structured "signs and symptoms" approach to patients with the following **clinical presentations** in developing countries including appropriate work-up, management, and follow-up based on available resources. *(Emphasis will vary depending on field of specialty):*

- Fever
- Respiratory distress
- Abdominal abnormalities, including pain, diarrhea and splenomegaly
- Anemia
- Skin abnormalities
- Under/severe acute malnutrition
- Jaundice
- Seizures and altered mental status

This list is not meant to be an exhaustive list, and would be country/region specific

OBJECTIVES:

1.   **Epidemiology/Public Health and Prevention:**

      a.   Describe the epidemiology, trends, and major causes of **infant, child, maternal, and adult mortality and morbidity** in developing countries, and contrast them with industrialized countries.

      b.   Recognize the **major underlying socioeconomic and political determinants of health**, and how these impact inequities in survival and health care access between and within countries.

      c.   Identify epidemiological trends and significance of **emerging infectious diseases** in the developing world.

      d.   Describe the impact of **environmental factors**, including safe water supply, sanitation, indoor air quality, vector control, industrial pollution, climate change, and natural disaster on health in developing countries.

      e.   Demonstrate a basic understanding of **health indicators** and **epidemiologic tools and methods**, and how they may be used in resource-limited settings to monitor and evaluate the impact of public health interventions for prevention and treatment of major diseases/conditions.

EPIDEMIOLOGY/PUBLIC HEALTH AND PREVENTION EXAMPLES

Pediatrics	Obstetrics & Gynecology	Internal Medicine
Describe the epidemiology of neonatal mortality, infant mortality and under-five child mortality. Compare and contrast common causes of mortality in each age group (neonatal, infant, under-five) according to region.	Recognize the leading causes of maternal mortality. Describe the model for the "three delays" in relation to maternal mortality. Recognize the impact of maternal mortality on infant and child morbidity and mortality.	Describe the leading causes of morbidity and mortality of adults in each major age group. Describe the role of emerging infectious diseases in contrast to morbidity and mortality of chronic diseases.
Identify prevention strategies specifically aimed at reducing neonatal morbidity and mortality. Describe known effective interventions for reducing under-five mortality and morbidity.	Describe the known effective interventions to prevent maternal morbidity and mortality in developing countries.	Describe effective interventions to prevent adult morbidity and mortality in developing countries. Describe effective interventions to diagnose and treat common adult presentations (e.g., IMAI).
Review the vaccine-preventable diseases and immunizations available in developing countries.	Describe the proportion of births normally attended by skilled personnel in developing countries.	Describe the impact of chronic diseases on the overall health, economic, and social sectors in the local region. Describe the incidence of trauma in adults, effective interventions and prevention strategies.
Describe the impact of the "Lost Generation" on raising children in an HIV-endemic society,	Describe contraceptive options, cultural influences, and contraceptive prevalence across different populations in developing countries.	Describe the incidence and prevalence of MDR-TB and HIV in the local region
The above should be interpreted as examples and are not all-inclusive.		

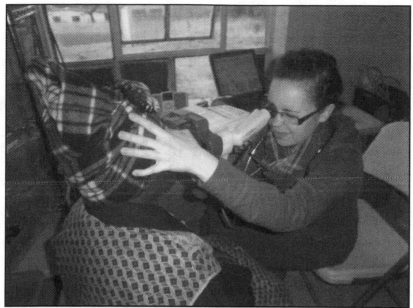

Using an autorefractor, first year Wright State University medical student
Alicia Boyd fits a patient in rural Swaziland with her first pair of eyeglasses.
(Photo credit: Megan Little.)

2. **Specific Conditions:**

a.   Recognize signs and contrasting features of chronic malnutrition, acute malnutrition and micronutrient deficiencies

b.   Describe and compare the different **anthropometric measures** used to diagnose malnutrition, and principles of **prevention and management** of malnutrition.

c.   Describe the **interaction between malnutrition/micronutrient deficiencies** and infectious diseases in infants, children, and adults.

d.   Identify conditions that contribute to **morbidity and impaired cognitive development** in the developing world such as intestinal parasites, hearing loss, birth complications, malaria, anemia, infections, nutritional deficiencies, injuries, and environmental toxin exposures.

e.   Describe the presentation, diagnosis, management, and prevention strategies of **infectious diseases** in resource-limited settings, based on local and international guidelines, including bacterial meningitis, dengue fever, diarrhea and dysentery, hepatitis A & B, HIV/AIDS, malaria, measles, pneumonia, polio, tuberculosis, typhoid fever, yellow fever, helminthic infections, and syphilis.

f.　　　Describe presentation, diagnosis and management of chronic diseases that contribute to adult morbidity and mortality, including hypertension, heart disease, cerebral vascular accident, and renal failure.

g.　　　Management of initial emergency presentations such as sepsis, trauma, and stroke.

SPECIFIC CONDITIONS EXAMPLES		
Describe the approach to the following issues and illnesses:		
Pediatrics	Obstetrics & Gynecology	Internal Medicine
Prenatal care in resource-poor settings Intrapartum fever, hemorrhage, complicated labor Prevention of mother-to-child transmission of HIV Neonatal resuscitation and care in resource-poor settings		Myocardial infarction, congestive heart failure, hypertension
Neonatal infections, including neonatal tetanus, sepsis, omphalitis, acute respiratory infections, etc.	Obstructed labor, maternal hemorrhage, intrapartum infection	Chronic obstructive pulmonary disease, chronic kidney disease, chronic liver disease, diabetes
Low birth weight infants	Ectopic pregnancy, complications from terminated pregnancies	Dementia, stroke, neuralgia
Acute respiratory infections, diarrheal diseases, fever	Hypertensive diseases of pregnancy	Cancer, paraneoplastic syndromes
Childhood injuries, including drowning, toxic ingestions, burns, and motor vehicle accidents	Female genital cutting, domestic violence, and sexual assault	Alcoholism, drug abuse, mental illness
The above should be interpreted as examples and are not all-inclusive.		

3.　**Specific Populations**
　　a.　　　Describe common health, social, and psychological issues faced by **immigrant and refugee populations** in developed nations.

b.   Describe health issues of people in the developing world affected by humanitarian crises, with particular attention to the problems of refugees, internally displaced persons, and orphans.

SPECIFIC POPULATIONS EXAMPLES		
Pediatrics	Obstetrics & Gynecology	Internal Medicine
Understand the health and psychological impact of child trafficking, child soldiers, and child labor.	Discuss issues of gender equity and major causes of inequality in women across different cultures in developing countries.	Describe how war or conflict has affected the mortality and morbidity of the community.
Identify specific health issues and needs of international adoptees, and describe appropriate screening and counseling for adopting families.	Identify the challenges for family planning in the region.	Estimate the approximate number of civilian deaths secondary to war in the region and the ratio between civilian and military casualties.
Understand the challenges faced by children living with disabilities in resource-poor settings, and describe prevention strategies and models of support.	Describe some challenges that are specific to pregnant women (barriers to recognition of medical emergency, inadequate health care services available, unsafe abortions, etc).	Describe how resettlement of refugees and asylees may shift epidemiology of mortality and morbidity of adults.
Identify medical priorities of displaced populations (vaccination campaigns, malnutrition, management of infectious and chronic diseases, obtaining clean water, etc.		
The above should be interpreted as examples and are not all-inclusive.		

Competency 3: Interpersonal Skills and Communication
Demonstrate interpersonal and communication skills that result in information exchange and partnering with patients, their families, their communities, and professional associates.

OBJECTIVES:

1.   Appropriately **utilize interpreters and communicate effectively** with families who speak another language.

2.   **Communicate effectively and respectfully** with physicians and other health professionals in an international setting, in order to share knowledge and discuss management of patients.

3. Develop **effective strategies for teaching** students, colleagues, and other professionals in settings with varying levels of knowledge or understanding of medical English.

4. Demonstrate awareness of **effective communication approaches** for delivery of health care and promotional messages in communities with **limited literacy and education**.

5. Familiarize yourself with **medical resources** that are available for **lay health care personnel** (e.g., community health workers, midwives, community leaders, lay counselors, etc.).

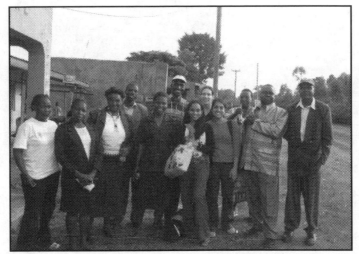

University of Pennsylvania global health track residents working with community health workers in Shibuye, Kenya. (Photo credit: Jennifer Cohn.)

Competency 4: Practice-based Learning and Improvement
Demonstrate knowledge, skills, and attitudes needed for continuous self-assessment, using scientific methods and evidence to investigate, evaluate, and improve one's patient care practice.

OBJECTIVES:
1. Identify **standardized guidelines** (e.g. WHO's Integrated Management of Childhood Illness - IMCI) for diagnosis and treatment of conditions common to developing countries and adapt them to individual needs of specific patients.

2.   Know and/or access **appropriate medical resources** and apply them to the care of patients in the developing country setting.

3.   Outline the principles of **evidence-based medicine** and apply them when reviewing recent literature and considering the implications for impact on practice.[1]

4.   **Work collaboratively** with health care team members to assess, coordinate, and improve patient care practices in settings with limited resources.

5.   Apply and improve upon **physical examination skills** and clinical diagnosis in settings where diagnostic studies are limited.

6.   Establish **individualized learning objectives** for an international elective and strategies for meeting those objectives.

7.   Describe your specialty's role in responding to **humanitarian emergencies and disaster relief efforts**, within the context of participating local and international organizations, and become familiar with available resources to prepare for volunteering in this setting.

Competency 5: Professionalism
Demonstrate a commitment to carrying out professional responsibilities, adherence to ethical principles and sensitivity to diversity when caring for patients in a developed or developing country setting.

OBJECTIVES:
1.   Demonstrate a commitment to **professional behavior** in interactions with staff and professional colleagues and be respectful of differences in knowledge level and practices.

---

[1] With the increasing focus on evidence based practice, adaptation of EBM resource-poor settings is an important component of a global health curriculum. The Cochrane Developing Countries Network (http://dcn.cochrane.org/en/localrevs.html) promotes research, practice, and access to health information and publications for developing countries. A method for integration of EBM into different branches of medicine is published online by Knowledge Translation (KT) Clearinghouse, found at http://www.cebm.utoronto.ca/syllabi/devl.

2.   Give examples of **cultural differences** relevant to care of international populations and how **traditional medicine** and Western/scientific medicine can conflict with or complement one another.

3.   Identify **common ethical dilemmas and challenges** confronted when working in a setting with limited resources or different cultural or ethnic values.

4.   Outline the **ethical standards and review processes for research** with human subjects carried out in developing countries, particularly involving vulnerable populations such as children and pregnant women.

5.   **Recognize personal biases** in caring for patients of diverse populations and different backgrounds and how these biases may affect care and decision-making.

6.   **Plan a responsible and ethically-guided international rotation experience**, ensuring adequate preparation and appropriate expectations both for yourself and your international hosts.

**Competency 6: Systems-based Practice
(Public Health Organization, Policy, and Advocacy)**
Understand how to practice high-quality health care and advocate for patients within the context of the health care system.

OBJECTIVES:
1.   Compare and contrast different **health care delivery settings in the developing world**, including hospitals, clinic and the community, and the roles of different health care workers as they apply to patients in developing countries, such as the physician, clinical officer, nurse, community health worker, and traditional birth attendant.

2.   Identify the **major governmental and non-governmental organizations** active in international health, and give examples of initiatives and programs that impact health. Understand how the policies and funding structures of these organizations as well as donor nations impact global health.

3.   Develop an understanding and awareness of the **health care workforce crisis in the developing world**, the factors that contribute to this, and strategies to address this problem.

4.   Identify different **health care systems and fee structures** between and within countries, including public and private sectors, and understand the impact of these systems on access to patient care and quality of care.

5.   Demonstrate sensitivity to the **costs of medical care** in countries with limited resources and how these costs impact choice of diagnostic studies and management plans for individual patients.

6.   Contrast the advantages and disadvantages of different approaches to implementing **health care interventions in developing countries**, such as vertical or targeted programs vs. integrated, focused vs. comprehensive, facility-based vs. community.

7.   **Advocate** for immigrant families who need assistance to deal with system complexities, such as lack of insurance, multiple appointments, transportation, or language barriers.

8.   Describe your specialty's role in **advocating for health policy** efforts that can reduce inequities and improve health of children and adults in developing countries.

SYSTEMS BASED PRACTICE EXAMPLES		
Pediatrics	Obstetrics & Gynecology	Internal Medicine
Describe the impact on policy, funding and program development of the following initiatives: - Millennium Development Goals -Global Fund for HIV, TB, Malaria - Roll Back Malaria - UN Rights of the Child	Describe the impact on policy, funding and program development of the following initiatives: - Millennium Development Goals - Safe Motherhood -Global Fund for HIV, TB, Malaria - Roll Back Malaria (maternal malaria)	Describe the impact on policy, funding and program development of the following initiatives: - Millennium Development Goals - Global Fund for HIV, TB, Malaria - Roll Back Malaria - WHO's List of Essential Medicines vs. National formularies
Describe strengths and weaknesses of:	Describe strengths and weaknesses of:	Describe strengths and weaknesses of:

- Integrated Management of Childhood Illness (IMCI) - Expanded Program on Vaccines (EPI) - Prevention of Mother-to-Child Transmission of HIV Guidelines - Severe Malnutrition Guidelines	- Expanded Program on Vaccines (EPI) - Prevention of Mother-to-Child Transmission of HIV Guidelines - Syndromic treatment of STDs Guidelines	- Integrated Management of Adult Illness (IMAI) -"Opt in" vs. "opt out" testing strategies for HIV
Describe the collaboration between different systems within the region (i.e. public health, medicine, and education).		
The above should be interpreted as examples and are not all-inclusive.		

Evaluation Tools

In addition to competency-based global health curricula and programming, residents may benefit from self-assessment tools such as a pre-trip fund of knowledge checklist. By taking the time to strengthen knowledge base in core areas prior to departure, a resident will better serve the host community and gain more from the international rotation. Below is an example of a list of core global health topics for a pediatric resident preparing to work abroad. This list can be adapted for any medical or surgical discipline. For example, the following checklist displays a "Fund of Knowledge Checklist for Pediatric Residents Working Clinically Abroad."

Diagnosis, Management, and Prevention of the Following Conditions According to Local and International Guidelines			
Infectious Disease		**Newborn Medicine**	
	Acute Respiratory Infections / Respiratory Distress		Routine Care of the Newborn
	Dengue Fever		Neonatal Resuscitation
	Diarrheal disease / Dysentery / Dehydration: - treatment of dehydration in setting of malnutrition		Low Birth Weight Neonates (hypoglycemia, hypothermia, intraventricular hemorrhages, seizure risk, sepsis)
	Diphtheria		Neonatal Infections (tetanus, syphilis, sepsis,

		HIV, HSV, etc)
	Fever (differential based on regional epidemiology, age, etc)	**Hematology**
	H. influenza related diseases (epiglottis, meningitis)	Anemia
	Hepatitis A, B & C	Sickle Cell Disease (vaso-occlusive crisis, splenic sequestration, fever management)
	HIV/AIDS and related infections / complications - management of HIV exposed infants - recognition of pediatric presentation of HIV (failure to thrive, chronic ARI, diarrhea, thrush, skin etiologies, etc)	**Neurology**
		Cerebral Palsy
		Seizures
		Altered Mental Status
	Malaria: - uncomplicated and complicated/severe (e.g. cerebral malaria) - first-line treatment guidelines based on region and resistance patterns	**GI / Malnutrition**
		Infant Feeding Guidelines
		Management of Severe and Moderate Malnutrition
		Micronutrient Deficiencies (Vitamin A, Zinc, Iodine, Iron)
		Fluid Management in Malnourished Children
	Measles	**Endocrine**
	Mumps	Diabetic Ketoacidosis
	Parasitic Infections (e.g. strongyloides, hookworm, amoebiasis, ascariasis)	Hypothyroidism
		Environmental
	Pertussis	Burn Management
	Polio (and sequelae)	Toxic Ingestions (including management of caustic ingestions in toddlers i.e. lye)
	Rubella	Envenomation
	Syphilis (neonatal and adolescent)	Smoke Inhalation
	Tetanus (neonatal and childhood presentations)	**Emergency Medicine (Pediatric)**
	Tuberculosis	PALS, NRP, preliminary airway management
	Typhoid Fever	Orthopedic Complaints (splinting, simple

		reductions)
		Trauma (including management of closed head trauma in varying age groups)
		Pneumothorax
	**Epidemiology / Public Health**	
	Identify major causes of child and infant mortality and morbidity	
	Identify major causes of maternal mortality	
	Identify effective interventions (e.g. breastfeeding, vitamin A supplementation, zinc supplementation, routine helminth treatment, ORS)	
	Identify major environmental hazards	
	Identify major priorities and challenges for children in Humanitarian Relief Settings	
	Identify options and resources for family planning, STI prevention and counseling	
	**Common Pediatric Global initiatives and Management Tools**	
	Describe the Expanded Program on Immunization (EPI)	
	Describe the Integrated Management of Childhood Illnesses (IMCI)	
	Describe the Prevention of Mother-to-Child-Transmission Guidelines (PMTCT)	
	Describe the Management of Severe Malnutrition (WHO)	
	Describe the Millennium Development Goals	
	Familiarize yourself with the national health system infrastructure: (role of community level centers, district/referral centers vs. NGOs)	
	Familiarize yourself with National Health Plans / Protocols supported by Ministry of Health of Host Country	

Competency-based Education: Implementation and Evaluation

The above suggested competency-based curriculum guidelines help define the content of global health education, based on the knowledge, skills, and attitudes residents are expected to develop in this field during a residency program. Developing objectives within the six ACGME competencies ensures that global health curricula move beyond the Knowledge/Patient Care domains and encompass others that may be overlooked, such as the Practice-based Learning and Professionalism domains. Having a defined set of curriculum guidelines such as those above can help guide both the program and the individual resident toward achieving well-defined, appropriate and realistic educational goals during residency, and should be used to guide program implementation as well as evaluation.

As suggested by the ACGME guidelines, it is important not only to consider the **content** of the individual objectives, but also the **setting** in which each objective will be learned. While there is obviously overlap between competencies within any method of teaching, the following suggestions regarding teaching methods are adapted from the ACGME Outcome Project:

- Objectives within the Knowledge and System-based Practice domains will likely be taught in didactic sessions, either lectures or discussions.
- Patient care objectives can be taught via lecture, as well as through case-based learning or direct clinical experience.
- Practice-based learning may occur through resident self-assessment or reflection on their experience.
- A journal club can be used to teach evidence-based medicine as applied to global health topics.
- Professionalism and Communication may best be taught through mentoring, role playing or case-based teaching.

In addition to "how" these objectives will be taught, the "where" of the setting becomes particularly important for global health curricula. Some objectives, such as developing knowledge about tropical diseases or immigrant health, may be more realistically achieved at the home institution, while others falling under the competencies of Professionalism, Communication and Practice-based Learning may be primarily learned through planning and experiencing an international elective rotation. Determining the "how" and "where" of competency-based learning is essential, not only for implementation but also for evaluation purposes.

The timing, or "when," of competency-based education may also be considered. Depending on the individual program, learning opportunities may be isolated to one brief educational activity such as a short course in tropical medicine or an international elective, or in the case of those programs with a longitudinal global health track learning may occur on a continuum over three years. Programs may further develop these competency-based objectives by determining which objectives will be achieved during the first, second and third years of residency, thereby providing further guidance for the individual resident. This can also lead to graded evaluation and self-assessment, providing different expected levels of achievement for the resident depending on their level of training.

Residents should be encouraged to familiarize themselves with the program's objectives and utilize them to develop their own individual objectives for a learning experience, particularly for planning an international elective. Development of individual objectives across a variety of competencies should be encouraged. For example, when planning an elective in a country in Sub-Saharan Africa, a resident could not only expect to learn about the clinical presentation and evaluation of malaria

(Knowledge/Patient Care), but also the international and local policies that drive malaria control strategies (Systems-based Practice), as well as application of standardized WHO guidelines to the management of this disease (Practice-based Learning). The knowledge checklist provided in this chapter can also be useful in guiding a resident's individual learning objectives.

The ACGME recommends various methods for evaluating resident learning and performance based on the six competencies. Some modalities commonly used in residency programs such as written examinations can be used in global health curricula to assess knowledge acquired through didactic teaching at the home institution. When considering the limitations of evaluating residents in the setting of an international elective, some modalities may be more feasible than others. For example, case logs may be a feasible evaluation method for Patient Care objectives and particularly valuable during an international elective. However, other recommended modalities such as the "360 degree" or "multi-rater" evaluation may be difficult or impossible due to the number of participants needed to give reliable evaluations and the likely effects of language and cultural barriers. Faculty mentors at the end of an international elective or residency program should apply the competency-based guidelines when developing evaluation tools for use. These evaluation tools will likely span all competencies. It may not be realistic to assess every curriculum objective, instead limiting assessments to a selected number of essential objectives. Examples of evaluation templates for resident international electives are included at the end of the chapter.

One challenge to applying competency-based guidelines to resident evaluation is that many objectives are best learned during the international elective, a time when evaluation is likely to be most difficult. An on-site faculty mentor may have insufficient opportunities to interact with a visiting resident or be inadequately trained in the proper use of evaluation methods. Similarly, focused one-time direct observations may be more time-efficient, but again lack of familiarity or training with these tools at the international site may make them less useful. At some programs the resident will be accompanied by a faculty mentor from their institution, but for most international electives this does not occur. A faculty mentor at the home institution would more likely be oriented to and familiar with standard evaluation tools, but would not be able to directly observe the resident during the international elective.

Because of these challenges, resident self-assessment and evaluation using the competency-based objectives may provide a useful adjunct to faculty evaluation. Residents can assess their competency at the beginning and end of the residency, or in preparation for and on completion of a rotation experience. A faculty mentor could then review and approve this evaluation tool, even though he or she may not have had the opportunity to directly observe them. A self-assessment scale such as one suggested on the APA Educational Guidelines Website can be applied to selected objectives:

What level of mastery do you feel you have achieved?

1 = none, just beginning
2 = limited experience, developing familiarity
3 = familiar, need more experience
4 = comfortable managing with limited guidance
5 = ready for independent practice

This type of self-assessment regarding the desired competencies is encouraged for the entire scope of a residency and not just for the global health competencies. Examples of resident self-assessment tools to be used for international electives as well as a didactic course are included at the end of this chapter. The role of faculty mentorship and feedback is of course essential to this process, and is addressed fully in Chapter 9.

Both faculty evaluation and resident self-assessment are limited by the lack of existing standards for the level of achievement residents should acquire for each competency in the field of global health. For example, based on the qualitative evaluation scale above it is reasonable to expect graduating residents to be "ready for independent practice" when managing the workup of a febrile patient in their home institution. Due to limited time spent overseas, the resident may only be expected to be "familiar" or "comfortable with providing care under limited guidance" in a developing country setting. The evaluation scale used should therefore be based on the individual residency program, extent of curriculum and expectations for the residents.

In addition to individual resident evaluation, utilizing assessment tools based on curriculum guidelines provides a format for global health program evaluation. Results over time of faculty evaluations, self-assessments or performance on written exams can be used to determine how well the program is meeting the designated objectives as well as identify areas of improvement. Program evaluation is covered comprehensively in Chapter 6.

To better understand the evaluation of competency in global health, we conducted a nonscientific survey of residency programs involved in global health. The mature programs had a curriculum in global health that was a standard part of residency teaching. Housestaff that were part of a global health track were provided additional lectures on topics such as cultural competency, humanitarian emergencies, global health policy, environmental health, and epidemiology. Many of the programs provide a week-long intensive course to these select global health residents and/or allowed them the opportunity to obtain a degree in public health or tropical medicine. Besides the standard international health elective abroad, stateside rotations, such as refugee health, tuberculosis/HIV clinic, and travel clinic, were integrated as part of the residency program. Unfortunately, the time and effort to create these global health programs and the limited engagement of faculty members have prevented the creation of national evaluation criteria for competency. Most directors and faculty members actively sought out qualitative feedback from residents and international health sites. However, very few have any standardized or validated evaluative tools on the international health site, the faculty, or the residents. The following section contains examples of competency-based evaluation tools that can evaluate the resident from multiple perspectives (self-assessment, faculty mentor and on-site mentor). These tools were designed for pediatric residents, and can be adapted to any field of medicine.

Pediatric Resident International Rotation Suggested Self-Assessment Tool *Adapted from Competency-based Curriculum Objectives*	Level of mastery <u>before</u> rotation	Level of mastery <u>after</u> rotation
What level of mastery do you feel you have achieved? 1 = none, just beginning 2 = limited experience, developing familiarity 3 = familiar, need more experience 4 = comfortable managing with limited guidance 5 = ready for independent practice	1 2 3 4 5	1 2 3 4 5
Apply and improve upon physical examination skills and clinical diagnosis in settings where diagnostic studies are limited.		
Demonstrate understanding of the presentation, differential diagnosis and management of pediatric patients with the following problems: • Diarrhea/dehydration • Respiratory Distress • Fever (including malaria) • Seizures/Altered Mental Status • Malnutrition (including Severe Acute Malnutrition)		

• HIV/AIDS (infection or exposure) • Tuberculosis • Burns • Newborn Care • Neonatal Resuscitation • Vaccine preventable diseases • Other (resident can fill-in site-specific goals):		
Demonstrate working knowledge of standardized guidelines (e.g., WHO/UNICEF) for diagnosis and treatment of conditions common to the setting (malaria guidelines, PMTCT, management of malnutrition, etc).		
Identify the top causes of neonatal and childhood mortality specific to the host country.		
Recognize underlying socioeconomic and political determinants of infant/child health specific to the local situation.		
Demonstrate an understanding of the health care delivery system in the specific setting, including, governmental and/or private hospitals, referral clinics and community level clinics.		
Demonstrate an understanding of the roles of different health care workers such as the physician, nurse, community health worker, traditional birth attendant, etc. as they apply to patients.		
Short Answer Questions:		
1. Identify a common ethical dilemma or challenge you confronted when working in a setting with limited resources or different cultural values.		

2. Describe an example of cultural difference relevant to patients at the international site and how traditional medicine and Western medicine can conflict with or complement one another.

3. Demonstrate with one measurable indicator how a positive difference was impacted on the host community.

Pediatric Resident International Elective Faculty Mentor Evaluation *(to be completed by Faculty Mentor about Resident)*	Scoring: 0 – Not observed 1 – Below Expectations 2 – Marginal 3 – Meets Expectations			
Medical Knowledge	*1*	*2*	*3*	*4*
Recognizes underlying socioeconomic and political determinants of infant/child health specific to the local situation.				
Describes the epidemiology, trends, and major causes of newborn, infant and child mortality and morbidity in the country/location of the rotation.				
Practice-based Learning and Improvement	*1*	*2*	*3*	*4*
Establishes individualized learning objectives for an international elective and strategies for meeting those objectives.				
Identifies and utilizes the resources needed to prepare for an international rotation or work in a less developed country.				
Identifies common ethical dilemmas and challenges confronted when working in a setting with limited resources or different cultural values.				

Demonstrates working knowledge of standardized guidelines (e.g., WHO/UNICEF) for diagnosis and treatment of conditions common to the setting.				
Identifies appropriate medical resources (books, articles, etc.) and applies them to the care of patients in the developing country setting.				

Professionalism	*1*	*2*	*3*	*4*
Plans a responsible and ethically-guided international rotation experience.				
Describes examples of cultural differences relevant to care of patients at the international site and how traditional medicine and Western/scientific medicine can conflict with or complement one another.				

Systems Based Practice	*1*	*2*	*3*	*4*
Demonstrates an understanding of the health care delivery system in the specific setting, including hospitals, clinics and the community.				
Demonstrates an understanding of the roles of different health care workers as they apply to patients, such as the physician, nurse, community health worker, traditional birth attendant, etc.				

Resident Evaluation for International Elective - Faculty Evaluation (To be completed by on-site mentor about resident)

Please complete the following evaluation for the resident completing a rotation at your site by checking the appropriate box for each objective. Please include any additional comments at below.

Scoring: 0 = Not observed; 1 – Did not satisfy expectation; 2 – Satisfied Expectations

Resident Performance Expectations:	**1**	**2**	**3**
Applies a logical and appropriate clinical approach to the care of patients in a developing country setting, utilizing locally available resources.			

73

Provides culturally sensitive care and support to patients and their families.			
Demonstrates sensitivity to the costs of medical care in countries with limited resources and how these costs impact choice of diagnostic studies and management plans for individual patients.			
Practices effective communication with families who speak another language and utilize interpreters appropriately.			
Works collaboratively with health care team members to assess, coordinate, and improve patient care practices in settings with limited resources.			
Demonstrates professional behavior in interactions with all staff and respect differences in knowledge level and practices.			
Demonstrates effective teaching methods for students, colleagues and other professionals.			

Comments:

Conclusion

The borders of our nations are becoming more and more porous. Hospitals and residency programs are seeing traditional "international" diseases in the United States. Conversely, residency programs are sending their trainees to care for patients and families in international settings. The proposed global health curriculum competencies, resident competency checklist, and evaluation tools included in this chapter are meant to be guidelines and should not be considered prescriptive. We encourage residency programs to adapt these resources as necessary to ensure their relevance to local and international circumstances. As global health and residency programs mature, these guidelines will undoubtedly change and evolve.

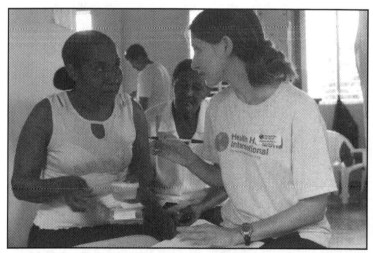

Laura McNulty, Executive Director of Health Horizons International, helps Francisca Garcia understand her treatment in the Pharmacy Education section of HHI's clinic in Severet, Dominican Republic. (Photo credit: Rachel Geylin.)

References

[1] Joyce B. Introduction to Competency-based Education: Facilitator's Guide. Accreditation Council for Graduate Medical Education (ACGME), 2006. Found on: Educating Physicians for the 21st Century: A 4-module educational resource for teaching and learning the competencies. www.acgme.org/outcome/e-learn/e_powerpoint.asp. Accessed 5/21/09.
[2] Kittredge, D., Baldwin, C. D., Bar-on, M. E., Beach, P. S., Trimm, R. F. (Eds.). (2004). APA Educational Guidelines for Pediatric Residency. Ambulatory Pediatric Association Website. Available online: www.ambpeds.org/egweb.
-- Allegrante J, Barry M, Airhihenbuwa C, Auld M, Collins J, Lamarre M, Magnusson G, McQueen D, and Mittelmark M. Towards Domains of Core Competency for Building Global Capacity in Health Promotion: The Galway Consensus Conference Statement, 2008 June.

-- Anandaraja N. Hahn S. Hennig N. Murphy R. Ripp J. The design and implementation of a multidisciplinary global health residency track at the Mount Sinai School of Medicine. Academic Medicine. 83(10):924-8, 2008 Oct

-- Baldwin, C, et al. Tutorial Modules 1-6. Based on: Kittredge, D., Baldwin, C. D., Bar-on, M. E., Beach, P. S., Trimm, R. F. (Eds.). APA Educational Guidelines for Pediatric Residency. Academic Pediatric Association (APA), 2004. Found at: www.academicpeds.org/egwebnew/index.cfm. Accessed 5/21/09 *(registration required)*

-- Houpt ER. Pearson RD. Hall TL. Three domains of competency in global health education: recommendations for all medical students. Academic Medicine. 82(3):222-5, 2007 Mar.

-- Penny S. Murray SF. Training initiatives for essential obstetric care in developing countries: a 'state of the art' review. Health Policy & Planning. 15(4):386-93, 2000 Dec.

Considerations in Program Development   5

Melanie Anspacher, Kevin Chan, Andrew Dykens Thomas Hall, and
       Christopher C. Stewart

An increasing number of residencies and fellowships are interested in developing global health programs for their residents and fellows. These programs confront many challenges and barriers: ensuring high-quality sustainable experiences with good mentoring abroad, finding salary support for residents traveling to other countries, and protecting the training program against liability risks. The central challenge is to build a high-caliber program without adversely impacting other aspects of the residency or of partner sites abroad. This chapter explores the hurdles and opportunities of developing global health programs and offers suggestions for addressing problems within individual institutions.

    For a newly developing or expanding global health program, it is important to conduct a background needs assessment within the home institution, identify key resources, involve key stakeholders in decision making early on in the process, develop supporters within relevant departments or schools, and garner support at the highest levels. For programs initiated by the leaders of the administration, this process may be easier, though arguing for sufficient resources to develop a quality program is often a challenge. When a program develops from the ground up, convincing administrators of the importance of the endeavor and the need for institutional support can be even more difficult. However, there are articles and experiences, outlined in chapter 1, which can be used to support the argument for developing, offering, and supporting global health programs. An excellent step-by-step book on curriculum development (not specific to global health,) is <u>Curriculum Development for Medical Education: A Six-Step Approach</u>, by David Kern, which breaks down the key steps in needs assessment and the support building process.[1]

    Curriculum development in a new and growing field such as global health is a complex task. Some immediate challenges include: setting achievable goals and objectives; identifying existing resources available to develop programs; incorporating global health teaching within current residency curricula and work hour requirements; and demonstrating the value of global health teaching. Successful curriculum development must ultimately rest on three cornerstones: a marked increase in knowledge about global health; enhanced skills in the provision of care in low-resource situations; and significant changes in attitudes and behaviors toward the provision of care to disadvantaged and marginalized populations.

Developing curriculum objectives

Global health program development is hampered by the lack of standardized guidelines for "good curricula". Program directors must decide whether to develop their own curricula or adopt and adapt existing curricula from other programs. The Accreditation Council for Graduate Medical Education (ACGME), through the Residency Review Committee, requires residency programs to develop competency-based guidelines. These guidelines can be useful in defining curriculum objectives across various areas of practice to ensure that global health curricula meet the same standards as other disciplines. Some examples of competencies for medicine and pediatrics can be found at: (www.acponline.org/fcim/index.html) and (www.ambpeds.org/site/education/education_guidelines.htm). Chapter 4 examines competencies in global health curricula.

Collaborating with medical education experts can expedite the process of high-quality curriculum development. Objectives developed by existing programs also may be used, such as those described in other chapters of this guidebook. Some objectives are appropriate regardless of specialty (for example, developing cultural competency), whereas others are specific to an activity (i.e. how to train local health workers in neonatal resuscitation).
Guidelines exist for global health as a supplementary learning experience. Some examples include pediatrics (via the Ambulatory Pediatric Association), and family medicine (www.aafp.org/online/en/home/aboutus/specialty/rpsolutions/eduguide).

Ideally, a program or curriculum in global health should include education about health and development issues in developing countries as well as a mentored international experience. Finding the time and resources within a residency program is challenging. Below are some suggestions that may be useful, along with obstacles that may be anticipated.

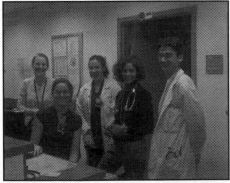

Members of the faculty, residency and NP training program at the East Baltimore Medical Clinic, part of the Johns Hopkins Urban Health Residency Program. (Photo credit: Rosalyn Stewart.)

Incorporating a Didactic Curriculum

The demand on residency programs to cover required topics and specialties limits the time for teaching about global health issues. As Chapter 2 indicates, a variety of methods of incorporating global health education into residency training are available. These include:

Protected teaching time: Topics in global health may be incorporated into protected conference time, including noon-time sessions and Grand Rounds, which are generally well attended. However, the number of global health lectures will likely be limited. "Institutional buy-in" (see below) is important to win the support of residency administration for the incorporation of global health topics.

Evening seminar series: Lectures, journal clubs, films, book discussions, etc., have been used to supplement residency activities in global health education. Resident work-hour requirements, however, have to be considered: institutions may decide that residents who stay longer hours to attend lectures violate their strict work-hour requirements, especially if these venues are a required part of the residency program. Family responsibilities and call schedules are other barriers to participating in evening sessions.

Elective time: Some institutions use elective rotations lasting from one to several weeks to provide training in global health. To reach the greatest number of participants with a superior course, consider partnering with other disciplines. While these will often be health science-related, consider also non-health related disciplines that have much bearing on global health such as anthropology, economics, engineering, politics, agriculture, international development studies, etc.

Self-study: Using web-based or computer-based modules and modular courses (see Chapter 8).

Field experiences: If faculty members accompany residents on their international experience, this may be the best time for focused, case-based teaching.

More than one strategy may be used to incorporate global health teaching into residency programs. Starting with a needs assessment of residents may help identify the best format to implement in a given program.

Ensuring Quality, Accountability, and Mentorship in Overseas Rotations

Many program directors ask for guidance in finding appropriate training opportunities for residents.   Ensuring that international electives are safe, academically accountable, and adequately supervised by individuals invested in teaching is extremely important, not only for the individual resident, but to guarantee the program's credibility and sustainability. Program directors, therefore, must carefully consider how these experiences will be offered to residents and evaluated.

The ideal mentorship system will link residents with faculty who are working abroad. The faculty mentor must have the time and commitment to supervise the resident properly. With this arrangement good mentoring is assured and the burden on host country faculty or staff is lessened. The faculty mentor can prepare a resident for the first global health experience and enrich the experience for a resident with previous experience abroad.

Other options to consider in establishing international partnerships:

Develop institutional relationships with international colleagues: This type of partnership may be either developed specifically for your program, or based on a previously established relationship. Detailed objectives, procedures and supervisory agreements for the rotation of residents should be developed collaboratively between the parties. Partners should collaborate in an ongoing evaluation process. A long-term, sustainable commitment promotes strong relationships with robust investment between partners home and abroad.

Identify individual partners: Individual partners within the community abroad, such as a local physician or practitioner can make a valuable connection to provide residents with appropriate supervision, teaching and feedback. Communication between the home institution and the abroad mentor and institution is essential and clear expectations set out ahead of time. Particular attention to communication such as spoken language, and phone/internet access must be taken into account. Building and nurturing relationships takes time. If possible, invite mentors to visit your institution to give them the opportunity to learn about educational models in North America, and to teach and exchange ideas on medical education.

Collaborate with another home country institution: Other institutions may have faculty traveling to a desired international site. Arrange for your resident to be mentored by that faculty member.

Develop formal evaluation processes with international partners: The evaluation process should include faculty, site, and program, as well as individual resident evaluation. Resident experiences should be evaluated by their supervisor and hosts, so it is important to ensure communication between sites.

Provide host country faculty with adjunct appointments at the resident's

<u>home institution:</u> This can be an excellent way to develop a partner relationship and to add prestige to colleagues abroad. This arrangement may take considerable resources and institutional commitment, but the rewards can be substantial. For example, the University of Toronto's Office of International Surgery invited an Ethiopian surgeon for a one-year fellowship to learn about medical education and surgery. He received an appointment as an adjunct professor at the University of Toronto. Within a year of his return to Ethiopia, he was named dean of medicine at his home academic institution. Adjunct professorship brings not only recognition, but also provides benefits such as online access to the medical school's library, accountability and opportunities for promotion. Providing small honoraria to partner faculty is a more modest way to help ease the cost/burden of a resource-poor country's faculty participation and to solidify relationships.

<u>Join existing international partnerships</u>: Association with existing programs may be more feasible than creating a new program, especially for small residency programs or those based outside large institutions. Many existing programs would like to provide a year-round resident or faculty presence at their international sites. Partnering locally and regionally may be an approach that builds a program's capacity.

Networks are being formed in South Asia, Latin America, and Africa that provide short-term medical education learning opportunities. Helping support international colleagues to acquire better skills to teach may help your residents in the long run. For example, the Essential Surgical Skills program in Ethiopia attracts surgeons and surgical assistants from Kenya and Sudan (www.cnis.ca).

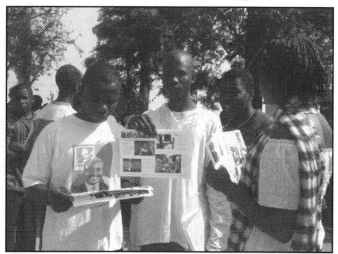

Mozambican students distribute newsletters on healthy living in their community. (Photo credit: Paul Johnson)

Performing Research Projects Overseas

Many residents who wish to conduct research may find the opportunity to perform projects abroad enticing. Residents researching abroad must remember this simple dictum: when research is done "on" a community, it must be "owned" by the community. The purpose of research is not just to enhance your curriculum vitae but to genuinely help your partner and communities abroad. So when a resident asks, "Should I do research overseas?" The response must be, "It depends."

Whether a research project is appropriate for an international venue depends on the relevance of the research question, the length of time available, and the accessibility of suitable mentors. Even in the best of circumstances, research is time-consuming to complete, and internationally-based research in the context of residency training is particularly difficult to achieve. Thus it is often best to have a resident work with a faculty member already doing research abroad. Such an arrangement may provide the additional benefits of conducting research relevant to the host country, developing closer relationships with host country faculty, and perhaps bringing residency-based research expertise and support to the aid of the host country researcher.

A resident with specific research questions in mind will need to begin planning early in residency, because it often takes two years to interest colleagues abroad, write the protocols, obtain funding, and gain final project approval. Before undertaking most research projects residents must get Institutional Review Board approval both at home and abroad. This process can take considerable time. Planning for delays and unforeseen circumstances is critical, and even the best plans may fail due to unforeseen circumstances. Residents should have proper training and guidance in planning and carrying out their project in an ethical and responsible manner. Chapter 3 discusses ethics of international work, including research, in detail. Co-authorship with host community partners should be strongly encouraged, if not required, and the parties should determine in advance their respective author roles if publication is likely. Having a local partner serve as lead author in a national journal (from the resident's home country) while the resident is lead author on a sufficiently different article in an international journal can be a useful way to recognize host country collaborators.

Given the short period allowed for most international electives and the time needed for visiting residents to learn community dynamics and establish relationships, independent research projects without long-term faculty presence or affiliation are difficult. Accordingly, residencies need to ensure adequate preparation and mentorship prior to incorporating overseas research into a global health curriculum.

While overseas research may be impractical, an ongoing service project, without a research focus, may provide a better fit with the global health program's goals or requirements. Examples of such projects include community needs assessment, education or training program development and implementation, public health infrastructural planning and construction, and clinic improvement projects. These activities can meet the expressed needs of local communities in ways that strict research may not, and can allow for sustainable work by multiple residents over time. Data collection, monitoring and evaluation of such projects can provide intrinsic research opportunities. The same principles of local ownership, involvement, and co-authorship should apply.

Many residency programs require that residents complete an academic project. Project examples, from a four to eight week U.S.-based program with international site mentorship, include: developing a simple assay in the clinic laboratory; producing an antibiogram for local hospital pathogens; teaching in a *promotora* (health worker) program; conducting a needs assessment in a local orphanage to promote health for the resident children; and assessing incidence of a particular disease in the community. Ideally, such a project teaches residents how to plan, carry out, summarize and present results. In addition, the results can contribute to the health of the local community. In contrast to formal research projects, academic projects may be more easily planned after arrival in the host country. Upon return to their host institution, residents may be required to present their project to peers or faculty.

Evaluating Global Health Programs

As in other aspects of residency and fellowship education, global health programs should be evaluated for their effectiveness. Evaluation measures should be built into the program from initiation, and refined with the acquisition of experience. Competency-based evaluation is discussed in detail in Chapter 4, ethics-specific evaluation in Chapter 3 and program evaluation in Chapter 6. Evaluation measures include monitoring participant changes in knowledge, medical and/or surgical skills, attitudes toward service, ability to communicate with patients, staff and community members, and career plans. The evaluation framework should take into account changes due both to experiences at the home institution as well as overseas. Demonstration of positive impact on resident education and compelling vignettes of program accomplishments are crucial in sustaining institutional support and funding.

Institutional Support

Support of the hospital and residency program is essential to the development and growth of a global health program. Support takes various forms: philosophical, personnel, and financial.

Gaining "institutional buy-in" is crucial to ensure from program initiation. Global health program faculty must demonstrate to hospital and residency program administrators that despite the barriers and costs, global health education is of great benefit to individual residents, to the residency program, and to international partners. In developing a proposal for a program, consideration may be given to the following factors:

Benefits to Resident Education:

● Global health education has a positive impact on the education and career choices of medical students and residents, stimulating interest in both academic programs and serving underserved and immigrant communities, as detailed in Chapter 1.

● Potential benefits of resident training in global health include improved physical exam skills, increased resource consciousness when making diagnostic and treatment decisions, experience working with underserved populations, increased interest in primary care, improved cultural competency, and increased first-hand exposure to working with medical issues that are uncommon in the US. [2,3]

● Residents gain significant experience addressing health disparities through developing skills in public health, community medicine, health advocacy, program development, economics, ethics, and service-based research. [4]

Benefits to Residency Programs:

● There is increasing interest in global health among medical students and resident physicians. In 1984, 6.2% of medical students participated in some form of international elective. [5] By 2007, 26.3% of students had worked abroad, [6] thus illustrating the potential draw, in terms of recruitment, to residency programs offering global health experiences. Miller et al., showed that 42% of applicants to Duke University's Internal Medicine Residency considered its global health programs an important factor in their selection. [7] Additionally, Dey et al. found that 68% of a sample of emergency medicine residents ranked programs with international opportunities. [8] In a study on the University of Colorado's Pediatric residency program, Federico et al. noted that 67% of the incoming intern class felt that international opportunities were important in the ranking process. [9] Bazemore et al. found that an international health track was the factor most strongly influencing choice of residency among family medicine applicants. [3]

● Global health programs create opportunities for faculty to advance clinical skills and participate in service-oriented practice, to the benefit

of faculty recruitment and retention.
- Residents who participate in global health experiences are more likely to practice among underserved and multicultural communities in the US as well as abroad. Residency programs may derive greater grant funding as the result of this practice selection.

- Global health activities provide opportunities for the development of research and scholarly activity both by home faculty as well as in conjunction with researchers abroad.

- Given the multidisciplinary nature of global health work, residency departments may collaborate with experts and institutions in public health, social work, environmental and infrastructural engineering, public policy, arts and humanities, education, water and sanitation, agro-forestry, pollution control and environmental preservation. Such collaboration could increase, profoundly, the richness of the department's mission while adding significantly to resources available within the community medicine curriculum.

- Global health activities demonstrate good will and unite the surrounding community toward the purposes of the institution's service, both domestically and abroad. Global health educational partnerships and service to international sites enhance the public image of medical schools and hospitals.

Benefits to Global Communities:

- Visiting faculty and resident physicians would be able to conduct short-term focused interventions such as providing clinical care or organizing other service-oriented activities. The visiting participants could, through close collaboration with the affiliated global community site, plan and/or provide supporting materials or equipment acquisition (with utmost consideration to appropriate technology). By explicitly educating residents prior to participation, a program could avoid offering services or medicines that might have a long-term negative impact while, offering some patient care that would have positive immediate impact and demonstrate good will.

- Visiting faculty and resident physicians would be able to participate within and support the local health system. As well, detailed community health education programs could be developed and implemented through their service.

- Partner health professionals may also benefit from the training capacity of the visiting resident's home institution, resulting in capacity building among individuals in under resourced communities. Such exchanges take place in stable partnerships and must consider sustainability and ethical considerations.

Accreditation Council for Graduate Medical Education (ACGME) Requirements

Accreditation Council for Graduate Medical Education requirements may complicate successful integration of experiences abroad into a residency program. The Resident Review Committee (RRC) for many specialties sets patient encounter and consecutive week quotas in clinics to ensure continuity. Residents traveling abroad often cannot meet these requirements for continuous care. Since this requirement is tied to funding from Medicare, one solution may be to fund resident slots independent of Medicare and to seek RRC exemption for global health pathways.

A related obstacle is the limited elective time available during a residency. Taking 1-2 months out of residency could be seen to detract from learning the basic competencies and limit the number of resident procedures required to define "competency," especially in surgical programs. Some programs have been successful in providing longer experiences abroad, either by RRC exemptions, or by creating flexible tracks in which residents can work abroad without credit towards residency requirements.

Minimizing Liability Risks

Many residency programs struggle to address liability risks arising from residents and their families traveling abroad and from litigation from patients in host countries. Residents may have to care for severely ill patients in situations where laboratory tests, x-rays, staff, and consultant support are inadequate. As in all patient care, some bad outcomes are unavoidable. To the present, liability cases have been very few in number and injury damage awards small – a situation that could change as more residents travel abroad for global health purposes.

Each program, in conjunction with its risk management or legal department, needs to develop policies and procedures, and make administrative support available to trainees abroad. Trainees should be aware of home institution policies and administrative support prior to departure.

Each program should provide pre-travel orientation for residents. This orientation should include: information and advice on expected and unacceptable participant behavior; personal health issues (including travel and safety advice, immunizations from a travel medicine clinic, and provision for emergency evacuation); contingency advice for commonly encountered problems; and provision for obtaining support in cases of adverse outcomes. The importance of discretion in matching clinical responsibility with current level of competence should be emphasized – an admonition that may be hard to honor when confronted with very sick patients in a low-resource situation. This issue is addressed in greater detail in Chapter 3, "Ethical Considerations for Global Health Residency Training."

Residents should be advised that if they do not follow guidelines they will be warned and may be removed from the project site. A faculty member or overseas site mentor should be given the authority to remove a resident.

Communication is also important. E-mail and mobile phones should be used whenever possible, and if consistent on-site mentoring is unavailable, residents should send brief progress reports to home institution mentors at agreed-upon intervals.

Global health training programs should ask residents who participate in abroad rotations to sign a waiver, acknowledging the risks of working and traveling abroad. Prior to departure, residents should also provide a one-page information sheet containing emergency contact information, travel plans, passport and visa information, and an affirmation that they have reviewed country information from the U.S.A. State Department web site (or the Department of Foreign Affairs and International Trade in Canada). This step should be implemented in pre-trip orientation, and the information sheet safeguarded by the residency program administration or the global health center. As part of the consent process, each resident should confirm having made provision for travel, health, and evacuation insurance. One good source of insurance is International SOS Insurance (www.internationalsos.com), but a number of other reputable companies are available. As a suggested guide, a minimum of $100,000 medical insurance coverage plus travel evacuation insurance should be provided. Universities may invest in services that track residents and provide safety warnings for trainees in areas threatened by armed conflict, natural disasters or other contingencies. The following pre-rotation guides may prove useful:

- Global Health Education Consortium (GHEC). The GHEC Guidebook: Advising Medical Students and Residents for International Health Experiences. (http://www.globalhealth-ec.org/GHEC/Resources/IHMECguidebk_resources.htm)

- Paul Drain, Steve Huffman, Sara Pirtle and Kevin Chan. *Caring for the World*. Toronto: University of Toronto Press (2009).

- Module 93 of the GHEC module project. (http://globalhealthedu.org/modules)

Impacts of Overseas Placements on Other Residents

Global health residency programs may find that residents not involved in the global health track are increasingly resentful of those who travel abroad, leaving them with heavier workloads and more frequent on-call schedules. Program directors will need to ensure that the on-call burden is equally divided among all residents throughout the year. The following are possible solutions:

- Residents are given "call-free" electives in which they travel abroad.

- Residents should "make-up" their lost call time due to overseas assignments

- With regard to continuity clinics, programs should establish policies with flexibility to allow residents to meet clinic requirements (especially in light of ACGME and RRC requirements,) and pursue an international elective. It is important to create an environment in which schedule changes are supported by administration, faculty, and residents; and where international experiences can enrich residency education for all learners, for example, by knowledge-sharing at post-travel conferences and presentations given by returning global health residents.

Obtaining Salary Support

A chief concern of residency program directors is obtaining funding to support resident salaries while abroad. Salary support is often tied to on-site services at home hospitals, and when residents/fellows travel abroad, the resulting shortfall in revenue makes it difficult to justify and support global health activities. Many programs seek and obtain independent support for resident international electives, either through discretionary departmental funds or by appealing to outside donors (individuals, medical alumni funds, or foundations). In some residencies, alumni classes have created endowments for a "global health residency position." One well-established relationship involves the Johnson and Johnson Foundation and Yale University. This program, known as the Physician Scholars in International Health, supports many resident international experiences (http://info.med.yale.edu/ischolar/). The Hubert Foundation has provided $5 million to Emory University to develop a global health in residency and public health initiatives. A more recent example at the University of Washington is a Bill and Melinda Gates Foundation grant which funds the development of residency programs in global health.

An associated problem is funding faculty interested in global health. Academic medical institutions in the U.S. utilize a wide range of funding approaches to support faculty involved in global health work. At most institutions, global health is not recognized as a route to promotion, so faculty may be reluctant to become involved. Ideally, to ensure the growth of global health expertise, increases in departmental funds, general endowments, or grant funds will be earmarked to support faculty development and appropriate administrative support. As more global health programs are developed, clear criteria must be established for the evaluation and promotion of faculty who spend substantial time in global health teaching, research and service.

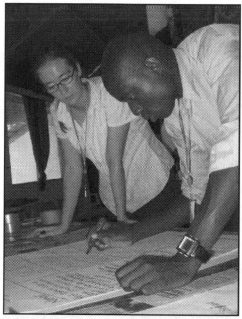

Elisabeth O'Brate works with community partners to plan health projects. (Photo credit: Paul Johnson.)

Family and Overseas Experiences

"Should I take my family abroad?" is a common question for residents planning to spend more than a few weeks away. Any family member who accompanies the resident while traveling should follow the same guidelines and requirements as the resident, as improper behavior could damage the relationship between host and home community, between academic institutions and between individuals. Family traveling abroad should accompany the resident for training and orientation to be aware of security, health, and welfare issues. Family members will need to make similar preparations regarding logistics, vaccinations, visas, and passports.

Residents who decide not to travel with the family will need to consider the implications for those who remain behind. This includes travel duration and expectations, communication arrangements, and support.

A "Global" View of Career Considerations

Living and working abroad has many life-enriching benefits. Even if an international rotation is short in duration, it can enrich the education and potential of a trainee in any field. However, there are career risks to keep in mind. Some employers will give credit towards career advancement for overseas experience, especially in government, academic and consulting organizations; while others may view time abroad as a negative, preferring that individuals advance their careers in home institutions. This may not be a serious consideration for those with a strong commitment to global health, especially those aspiring to a lifetime global health career. However, individuals with both aspirations in highly competitive fields and an interest in global health may need to consider the balance of positive and negative career effects of international work. Timing of international work (early in a career, or after establishing a successful practice,) family (greater enjoyment in working abroad prior to starting a family, or accompanied by a partner, spouse, or children), and ability for career support and advancement in a home institution while working internationally (by professional publications or periodic returns, for example) are all important considerations. While health professionals may face difficult choices between high levels of achievement in home institutions and the freedom to pursue global health work, increasing recognition of the universality of global health concepts and skills will inevitably lead to greater opportunities and wider interest among highly-resourced institutions.

Obtaining Non-salary Support

There are other costs to consider when setting up global health programs abroad: travel costs, including plane tickets and in-country travel, visas, passports, travel insurance and vaccinations. These costs can be substantial, especially in sub-Saharan Africa and South Asia. The two most common sources of funding for residents are families and churches or other religious organizations. Consideration should be paid to the effects of secular funding on health ventures, both in terms of ability to provide a spectrum of services as well as the cultural and religious context of the host community. As a final challenge, in the spirit of equality, programs might consider targeting travel funding support for international electives to residents with fewer resources so that global health experiences are not limited to the more affluent.

    A number of institutions seek support from outside donors (such as medical alumni funds or foundations). Some competitive fellowships can also help support travel abroad. These include the following, (as well as additional resources found in Chapter 8):

- Yale Johnson and Johnson Physician Scholars in International Health: provides a travel award ranging for $1,000-$5,000 (http://info.med.yale.edu/ischolar/description.html)
- MAP International Medical Fellowship: provides 100% of approved round trip airfare to one destination (must spend a minimum of 6 weeks) (www.map.org/site/PageServer?pagename=what_Medical_Fellowship)
- Rotary Foundation Ambassadorial Scholarship (www.rotary.org/foundation/educational/amb_scho?prospect/index1)
- American Medical Women's Association Overseas Assistance Grant (up to $1500) (www.amwa-doc.org)
- Christian Medical and Dental Association Johnson Short-Term Mission Scholarship (http://www.cmda.org/AM/Template.cfm?Section=Johnson_Short_term_Missions_Scholarship)
- Sara's Wish Scholarship Fund: For young women, pursuing the ideals of bettering the world (ranging from $1,000-$1,500) (www.saraswish.org)
- American Academy of Pediatrics International Child Health Travel Grant ($500)
- Canadian Paediatric Society International Child Health Grant ($750 Can)

References

[1] Curriculum Development for Medical Education: A Six-Step Approach. David E. Kern, Patricia A. Thomas, Donna M. Howard, and Eric B. Bass; The Johns Hopkins University Press, Baltimore, 1998.

[2] Evert J, Bazemore A, Hixon A, Withy k. "Going Global: Considerations for Introducing Global Health into Family Medicine Training Programs." (Fam Med) 39, no. 9 (2007): 659-665.

[3] Bazemore AW, Henein M, Goldenhar LM, Szaflarski M, Lindsell CJ, Diller P. "The effect of offering international health training opportunities on family medicine residency recruiting." (Fam Med) 39, no. 4 (2007): 659-83.

[4] Furin J, Farmer P, Wolf M, et al. "A novel training model to address health problems in poor and underserved populations." (J health Care Poor Underserved) 17, no. 1 (2006): 17-24.

[5] Panosian C, Coates TJ. "The new medical "missionaries"--grooming the next generation of global health workers." (N Engl J Med) 354, no. 17 (2006): 1771-3.

[6] Association of American Medical Colleges, Washington D.C. "2007 Medical School Graduation Questionnaire: all schools report." 2007. http://www.aamc.org/data/gq/allschoolsreports/2007.pdf (accessed July 16, 2008).

[7] Miller WC, Corey GR, Lallinger GJ, Durak DT. "International Health and Internal Medicine Residency Training: The Duke University Experience." *The American Journal of Medicine.* September 1995; 99: 291-297.

[8] Dey CC, Grabowski JG, Gebreyes K, et al. "Influence of international emergency medicine opportunities on residency program selection." (Acad Emerg Med) 9, no. 7 (July 2002): 679-83.

[9] Federico SG, Zachar PA, Oravec CM, Mandler T, Goldson E, Brown J. "A Successful International Child Health Elective: The University of Colorado Department of Pediatrics' Experience." *Archives of Pediatrics and Adolescent Medicine.* 2006; 160: 191-196.

Sophie Gladding, Cindy Howard, Andrea L. Pfeifle, and Yousef Yassin Turshani

Introduction - Importance of evaluation

In the global health education community, many professionals decided on their career paths based on international elective experiences during residency. Often residents and faculty alike will comment on how much they gained professionally and personally from their medical experience abroad. It is not unusual to hear a resident comment after an international elective, "It has changed my life forever and I have only become a better physician." What was the change? How did it happen? Is the resident really a better physician? Can this experience be duplicated at home for all residents even those who cannot go abroad? These are only a few of the questions to be asked and answered by graduate medical education programs committed to providing excellent training in global health. The answers will be found through evaluation of program outcomes.

The recent advent of global health tracks within residency curricula has generated much discussion about curriculum design and delivery, and focused attention on establishing international educational partnerships. In addition, in 2004, the Accreditation Council for Graduate Medical Education (ACGME)[2] mandated that all graduate-level training programs change to a competency-based process of education with a focus on outcome measures. This standard applies to training in global health as well. There is, therefore, a strong need for evaluation to document the outcomes of global health programs.

While there are ample anecdotes to demonstrate the benefits of global health programs, undertaking systematic program evaluation provides stronger evidence about the effectiveness of global health programs – critical to the success and sustainability of these programs. Evaluation can provide valuable information about whether a program is achieving its goals, identify what aspects of the program are working well, and generate suggestions for ways to improve.

Purpose of the evaluation

The first step in any program evaluation is to determine the purpose of the evaluation. Generally speaking, there are two types of evaluation: formative and summative. Formative evaluations are generally conducted

---

[2] The ACGME is a private, non-profit council that evaluates and accredits medical residency programs in the United States.

during program development, with the explicit purpose of guiding program improvement initiatives. Formative evaluations typically provide information about what is working and what needs improvement. Summative evaluations, on the other hand, are generally conducted once a program has been established. Summative evaluations typically describe the value of results or outcomes of the program in relationship to established criteria, such as the ACGME competencies. Formative evaluations often lead to program modifications while summative evaluations generally lead to decisions about program continuation, expansion or termination.

Formative evaluations address	Summative evaluations address
What aspects of the program are working? What aspects of the program need improvement? How can the program be improved?	What outcomes were achieved? By whom? Under what circumstances? At what cost?

Adapted from Worthen B.R. , Sanders, J.R. & Fitzpatrick, J.L. (1997). *Program Evaluation: Alternative Approaches and Practical Guidelines* (2nd ed). White Plains, NY: Longman.

Defining Program Structure and Goals

After determining the primary purpose of the evaluation, the next step is to clearly identify the goals and objectives of the program and describe how the components of the program (the curriculum, program activities, international elective, etc.) are expected to lead to the specified outcomes of the program. This can be diagrammed in a "logic model" that illustrates the links between program components and outcomes, for example:

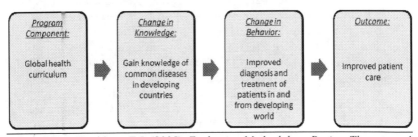

Adapted from Davidson, E.J. (2005). *Evaluation Methodology Basics: The nuts and bolts of sound evaluation.* Thousand Oaks, CA: Sage Publications.

Identifying stakeholders

After the purpose of the evaluation has been determined and the logic model defined, it is important to identify the stakeholders – all of the individuals and groups who have an interest or investment in the program outcomes. Thorough identification of stakeholders ensures that all relevant perspectives and concerns are included in the design of the evaluation. An example is found below:

Stakeholder	Concerns
Director of global health program	*Is the global health program providing an academically sound and safe experience for the participants?* *Are the international sites providing residents with an appropriate and safe experience?*
Global health program faculty members	*Is there sufficient time to mentor residents?* *Is there sufficient time to design and teach the global health curriculum?* *Is there funding to support the global health activities?*
Residency program director	*Is the global health program providing an academically sound and safe experience for the participants?* *Does the global health program support the curricular objectives of the residency program?* *Does the program attract strong residents to the residency program?* *Is there sufficient reimbursement to the residency program if there is an international health elective?*
Department chair	*Is there sufficient revenue to support the program?* *Does the global health program fit within the overall mission of the residency program?* *Is the global health program providing an academically sound and safe experience for the participants?*
Residents	*By the end of the program will they be able to care for patients in and from the developing world?* *Will there be a faculty mentor and international opportunity related to their particular area of interest?* *Will participation in the program enhance or detract from their career choices?*

	How will residents include the global health program into their busy residency schedule?
International elective on-site faculty members and staff	Are the residents well prepared for their experience abroad both medically and culturally? Will the presence of residents enhance or detract from the delivery of patient care?
Patients and families	Are residents and graduates of the program sufficiently trained to care for them or their family member? Are residents and graduates of the program able to communication effectively with them and their family members?

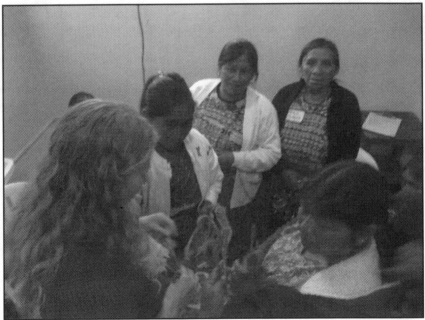

A group of Guatemalan traditional birth attendants teach UCSF CNM student and Global Health Clinical Scholar Kari Radoff about traditional herbal medicines. (Photo credit: KC Bly.)

Evaluation Questions

Once the program's goals have been defined and the stakeholders' concerns outlined, the central evaluation questions can be formulated. These questions, as in the examples below, should gather information about the extent to which program goals are being achieved and should also reflect stakeholder concerns.

Formative evaluation questions:

1.   To what extent does the content of the global health program curriculum cover the critical health care issues affecting patients in and from the developing world ?

2.   To what extent does each of the components of the program meet the needs of the residents?

3.   To what extent does each of the components of the program enhance or detract from the overall quality of the program?

4.   What are the effects of participating in a global health program in regards to increasing residents' knowledge of health care issues affecting patients in and from the developing world and delivering patient care that is culturally competent?

Summative evaluation questions:

Long-term impact of program:

1.   To what extent are graduates of the global health program involved in global health care after 5, 10 and 15 years?

Change in residents' knowledge:

2.   To what extent are participants able to demonstrate:
   a.   Medical knowledge of common diseases in the developing world
   b.   Knowledge of the causes and consequences of health disparities

Change in residents' skills:

3.   To what extent are participants able to demonstrate:
   a.   Patient care that is culturally competent
   b.   Cross-cultural interpersonal and communication skills with health care teams in international settings

Change in residents' attitudes:

4.   To what extent are residents and graduates engaged in working with under-served patient populations?

5. To what extent are residents and graduates involved in advocacy?

Determining Data and Evidence Needed

After the central evaluation questions have been established, the evidence or data needed to answer the questions and the sources of the data must be determined. Some of the data may already exist while other data may need to be collected. When making this determination, it is important to consider the relative ease with which the data will be accessed or collected and whether or not this can be accomplished within a reasonable timeframe and with available resources. The type of data or evidence collected must also be sufficiently compelling to convince stakeholders and decision-makers about the value of the program. Examples of possible types of data include Assessment of residents' knowledge, skills and attitudes: (the ACGME offers suggestions and examples of assessments for each of the ACGME general competency domains at http://www.acgme.org/Outcome/). See also Chapter 4.

- multiple choice tests of knowledge
- oral examination
- OSCE
- standardized patient examination
- direct observation by faculty members
- structured journaling/portfolio
- residents' self-assessment
- patient surveys
- 360 evaluations
- academic project

Residents' evaluations of program components and overall program assessment:
- surveys
- interviews
- focus groups

Longitudinal tracking of residents after graduation:
- surveys
- interviews

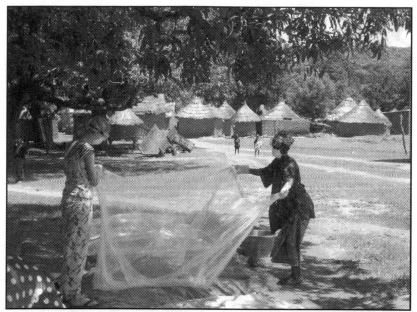

Mariel Bryden, medical student at the University of Iowa Carver College of Medicine, and community health volunteer Masakuru Keita lay a permethrin-treated bed net out to dry in Nana Kenieba, Mali. This bed net distribution project is sponsored by the NGO Medicine for Mali. (Photo credit: Benjamin Bryden.)

Setting Standards to Determine Success

Programs in global health must establish standards or specific criteria for assessment. The outcomes of the program can then be judged against the established standards.

These standards can either be absolute or relative standards. Absolute standards describe a set level of performance to be achieved by program participants. Absolute standards can be set by looking to established standards in the field or in the literature, or they can be set by the program by building consensus about the necessary level of performance with the program stakeholders.

Examples of absolute standards:

- Set levels for required attendance at noon conference, journal club, etc.
- Set levels of achievement on assessments of residents' performance (e.g. 80% of residents must achieve 90% or better on the knowledge test of global health)

99

Where differences in levels of performance are more important than absolute levels of performance, relative standards can be used. Relative standards are based on comparisons of performance either between groups or pre- and post- for a single group. Statistical significance or effect size, a measure of the size of the difference between two groups, is often used as the benchmark for relative standards.

Examples of relative standards include:

- Statistically significant difference between participants in global health program and non-participants in demonstrating culturally competent care
- Statistically significant difference between pre- and post-educational activity assessments for single group of residents in knowledge of global health issues.

Evaluation plan

The overall plan and structure of the evaluation is determined by the above steps and will guide the execution of the evaluation, as in the following example:

Evaluation Question	Data Needed to Answer Question	Sources of Data	Methods/ Strategies/ Analysis
Formative: 1. To what extent does the content of the global health program curriculum cover the critical health care issues affecting children in and from the developing world?	Content of the curriculum, including computer-based presentations or lecture notes from all relevant conferences (noon conferences, Grand Rounds, evening seminars, etc.), and web modules	Faculty members and guest lecturers in global health program	Expert content review – have all elements of the global health curriculum reviewed by several external experts in global health
Summative: 2. To what extent are participants	Performance-based assessment of residents' patient care and	Residents	Faculty evaluation of patient care and communication skills of residents both in country and on

able to demonstrate: a. Patient care that is culturally competent? b. Cross-cultural interpersona l and communicat ion skills with health care teams in international settings?	communication and interpersonal skills		international rotation OSCE with stations focusing on cross cultural communication skills and patient care of diverse patient populations
Summative: 3. To what extent are graduates of the global health program involved in global child health care?	Career paths and global health involvement of graduates of the program	Graduates of global health program	Longitudinal survey conducted every 5 years

Question of causation – evaluation design

An important question that is often asked in program evaluations is whether there has been a change in residents' knowledge or performance. Program providers and funders want to know if their program is working, how it is working, and whether specific changes that have been reported can be attributed to participation in the program.

While these are important questions, they are also often difficult questions to answer with certainty. Residents are learning and developing skills in a dynamic multi-factorial environment (the global health program, the general residency program, clinical rotations, their own independent learning, etc.) It is, therefore, often difficult to attribute gains residents make in knowledge, skills and attitudes specifically to the global health program.

Additionally, because residents choose to participate in global health programs, there is an issue of "selection bias" which may make it difficult to determine whether learning outcomes are due to the global health program (the intervention,) or are due to the characteristics of the residents who choose to participate in global health programs. Selection bias, therefore, poses a threat to the internal validity of the results of the evaluation. For example, if a larger percentage of participants of global health programs choose careers in primary care than non-participants, it is tempting to conclude that participation in global health programs leads to greater participation in primary care careers. It is, however, not possible to know, without further investigation, whether this career choice reflects the influence of the global health program or that residents who choose to participate in a global health program are also more likely to choose a career in primary care.

The first step in addressing the question of causation is to determine what level of certainty is needed regarding the attribution of outcomes to the program. It is generally the case that higher stakes decisions require greater certainty about causation. Formative evaluations often require a lower level of certainty about causation, while summative evaluations, which may affect the continuation of a program, demand a much higher level of certainty.

If a higher level of certainty about causation is needed, there are a number of evaluation designs or methodologies that can help to address the question of causation and reduce the threat of selection bias.

The only design that allows for causal claims to be made and controls for selection bias is an experimental design with random assignment (random controlled trial). However, this is not likely to be possible in global health programs where residents have autonomy regarding participation.

As random assignment is likely not possible, a more appropriate alternative might be a quasi-experimental design with a comparison group. In this design, there is not random assignment to the program, but outcomes of the program participants are compared with a nonequivalent control group of non-participants. For example, pre and post-test scores of participants and non-participants on a specific assessment (OSCE, written exam, etc.) could be compared using the appropriate statistical test (t-test, Chi Square, etc.) to determine whether there is a difference between the outcomes of the two groups and whether the difference is significant. As there is no random assignment is this design, selection bias is a real concern. This concern can be addressed to some degree by matching the participant group and the non-participant group on as many observable characteristics as possible, such as years of training, USMLE scores, in-training examination scores, etc. Greater similarity of the two groups based on observable characteristics creates a stronger argument that differences in scores between the two groups are differences due to participation in the global health program, as opposed to differences in characteristics between the two groups. Statistical regression analysis, using all of the observable characteristics in the model, may be conducted in order to control for extraneous variables so that any difference in the group outcomes are not due to the extraneous factors. A more extensive discussion of quasi-experimental designs can be found in Cook and Campbell (1979)[1] and further information about statistical analysis in Howell (2007)[2].

One commonly used design is a single-group design with a pre- and post-test comparison. This type of design measures change, but it is a weaker design in addressing the question of causation. For example, if a single group of residents participating in a global health program is pre- and post-tested on demonstrating culturally competent patient care, this would provide evidence about whether there was a change in residents' skill level, but it would not be possible to attribute this change to the global health program because the change could be attributed to another event such as training on culturally competent patient care provided to all residents as part of the general residency program.

The weakest design is a single group post-test only, design in which residents might be assessed at the end of the global health program. This type of design shows that outcomes have or have not been achieved. It does not measure change and does not provide evidence of causation.

In cases where only the weaker designs are possible, the size of the sample is insufficient for statistical analysis, or a lower level of certainty about causation is acceptable, there are a number of approaches to infer causation. These approaches require considerable interpretation and generalization in order to argue that observed changes are likely due to the global health program and to rule out other possible sources or causes.

Davidson (2005) suggests the following strategies for inferring causation:

- Asking participants about the cause
- Checking whether the content of the program matches the outcome
- Looking for and "ruling out" other possible causes
- Checking whether the timing of the outcomes makes sense
- Examining whether the response matches the dose
- Examining underlying causal links

In the evaluation of global health programs, these strategies could be operationalized in the following ways:

Asking participants: In this straightforward strategy, participants could simply be asked whether they thought that changes in their knowledge, skills and attitudes were caused by participation in the global health program or by other factors

Checking whether the content of the global health program matches the outcome: the content of the program should be reflected in the measured outcomes, in order for the program to be the cause of the outcomes. For example, if participants in the global health program improve their knowledge about global health disparities, which is an important content area in the program, then a reasoned argument could be made that participation in the program has led to the improved knowledge, particularly if other possible causes of gains in this content area could be ruled out (e.g. it is not a part of the general residency program).

Looking for and "ruling out" other possible causes: it is important to explore other possible causes of change observed in the residents. For example, it would be important to determine whether the changes observed in global health residents could be explained by participation in the general residency program. This question could be explored by examining whether the changes or patterns in the changes in global health residents are similar to residents not participating in the global health program. If the patterns of change are similar, this would suggest that the changes may be due to participation in the general residency program as opposed to the global health program.

Checking whether the timing of the outcomes makes sense: The argument for inferring causation can be strengthened if the timing of the outcomes is consistent with what would be expected from participation in the program. For example, in a hypothetical program, understanding the cultural practices around disease treatment is a focus of the second year of a program. If both first and second year residents are assessed at the end of the year in this area and second year residents show greater knowledge in this area than the first year residents, then this would strengthen the argument for inferring causation. Changes that are not consistent with the expected timing of outcomes might suggest that the outcomes could be due to another cause.

Examining whether the response matches the dose: In global health programs where there are multiple components in which residents can participate, there is an opportunity to examine whether the response (outcome) matches the dose (amount of participation.) This is to say, if residents participate in more of the components, one would expect that those residents would show greater gains than those who participated in fewer components of the program.

Examining underlying causal links: this can be a particularly useful strategy for examining distal outcomes such as career choice of graduates of global health programs. This strategy presents evidence of the series of links that logically connects the global health program with outcomes, thus strengthening the argument for inferring causation. For example, a program might hypothesize that participation in their global health program leads to future career involvement with under-served patient populations by their graduates. The hypothesis might be based on a series of causal links: (a) participation in the global health program leads increased knowledge about causes and consequences of health disparities; (b) improved knowledge of disparities creates greater sensitivity to the needs of under-served populations; (c) this sensitivity increases motivation to work with under-served populations. If evidence could be found for each of these links, this would support the argument for the causal relationship between participation in a global health program and subsequent work with under-served populations.

The strategy or combination of strategies that a program uses to infer causation is determined by the level of certainty needed, the accessibility of data and the availability of resources.

Evaluation questions that focus on perceptions and levels of satisfaction about the program, which are often important in formative evaluation, can be answered using descriptive designs. Instead of addressing questions of causation, these designs describe the programs being evaluated. For example, if a program seeks to assess resident satisfaction with a global health program and if the program meets their needs, a cross-sectional design could be used to survey residents about their attitudes regarding the program. Alternatively, the program could collect similar data via interviews or focus groups in order to describe residents' perceptions of the program.

Conclusion

Useful program evaluation as outlined above will require collaboration among all key stakeholders. Both home and host nation individuals and communities, including faculty members, residents and patients, will need to participate in the evaluation process. Global health programs require the collaboration and shared commitment of both the home institution and international partners in all aspects of the program, including the evaluation process. Establishing the key outcomes to be measured and the methods of evaluation will provide a structure by which residency programs can accurately determine achievement of the desired outcome. If data show that physicians become better equipped professionally and personally via global health educational programs, then the time commitment and funds needed to provide such training will follow.

References

[1]Cook, T.D. & Campbell, D.T. (1979). *Quasi-experimentation: Design and analysis issues for field settings.* Chicago, IL: Rand McNally.
[2] Howell, D.C. (2007). Statistical Methods for Psychology (6th ed.). Belmont, CA. Thomson Wadsworth.
-- Davidson, E.J. (2005). *Evaluation Methodology Basics: The nuts and bolts of sound evaluation.* Thousand Oaks, CA: Sage Publications.

-- Worthen B.R. , Sanders, J.R. & Fitzpatrick, J.L. (1997*). Program Evaluation: Alternative Approaches and Practical Guidelines* (2nd ed). White Plains, NY: Longman.

Lisa L. Dillabaugh, Daniel Philip Oluoch Kwaro, Hannah H. Leslie,
Jeremy Penner, and Sophy Shiahua Wong; with contributions from
S.M. Dabak, S.S. Dabak,, German Tenorio, and Wilfredo Torres

Rotation Planning

Part 1 - Choosing a site

Undertaking a global health rotation is often described as an incredible, life-changing experience. With an open mind and heart, rotations abroad can give the opportunity to more deeply understand the human condition. For many of us living in North America, a global health rotation is also a humbling experience. Working in communities abroad helps us to realize that we are all doing the best we can in the circumstances we are given, no matter where in the world we live.

Each site is unique. The following are some issues to consider when you are looking into global health programs.

A. Institutional Considerations (school and/or residency program)

- If you want or need credit, verify which programs are recognized by your school or institution. It will help you narrow down your choices quickly.
- If other students or residents have gone to a site which you are interested in the last one to two years, ask them about their experience. Consider your priorities between specific geographic locations, particular individual objectives, and recommendations of a program site by other students and residents. It is likely that you may have to balance these priorities.
- Assess the institutional presence at sites you are considering. Even if other students or residents have not completed rotations there, you may be able to identify research collaborations or other partnerships at the site that can provide useful information or an existing framework for collaborative activities.
- Find out if your institution will cover some of the costs (e.g. a special fellowship fund for certain sites, housing at an affiliated university's dorm, or a small stipend for rotation-related expenses.)
- Find out if your institution has any travel scholarships, global health fellowships, or related research grants.

B. Site Considerations: Geography and Safety

- Do you want to be in a specific region?
- Do you want to be able to speak a language largely spoken in that site?
- Check the CDC travel advisory website for the sites you are interested in. Is it safe to travel and live there for a short period of time?
- The US State Department also has a country-specific "Warning List," but keep in mind that this website may not reflect the true risk of the specific location or community where you will be. If the site you want to go to is on the list, check with your institution about whether or not it will allow you to go there. Many institutions will not provide funding for work in countries on the State Department Warning List.
- Have an open discussion with your family and your institution, to ensure that all are able to tolerate the risks of the sites you are interested in.
- Be flexible. Remember that unexpected risks, such as disease outbreaks, natural disasters, and political unrest can happen anywhere and at any time. Keep your options open and explore multiple sites in case of sudden changes. International travel can sometimes be unreliable. *You may need to go to Plan C if Plan A and Plan B don't work out.*

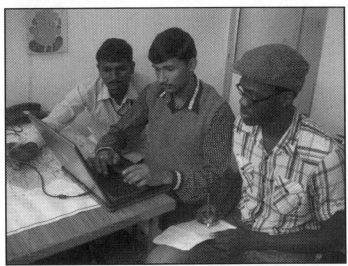

Ben Thomas (UCSF School of Medicine) working with public health outreach workers at Swami Vivekananda Youth Movement in Saragur, India to develop a map of the service area. (Photo credit: Katherine Holbrook.)

C. Program Considerations

There are a variety of programs offering or supporting global health rotations. These range from existing collaborations between academic institutions to organizations designed to provide international electives for a fee. Individual students and residents also set up rotations directly with clinics or hospitals abroad. When evaluating these options, consider your objectives for the rotation. The clearer your objectives are, the better the experience is likely to be.

- Do you primarily want a language program, a clinical site, or a site where you can conduct a research project?
- Do you want to be at an academic, community-based Non-Governmental Organization (NGO), or religious site?
- Do you want to be immersed in the community? Or primarily at an academic institution?
- Does your home institution or fellowship require you to perform a project in order to fulfill rotation requirements? If so, can the site you have chosen accommodate such a project? Will you have academic support and access to research materials at the host site? Will you have sufficient time to complete your project?
- What kind of roles and responsibilities do you want to have? Are these available in the site which you are considering?
- Do you want to go with a group or as an individual?
- Do you want to work independently or with more structure and pre-planned activities?
- Do you want to work or live with other visitors to the host community? (e.g. visiting students, residents, researchers, scholars)
- How much time do you have available? Many rotations are constrained by residency restrictions. Consider what you can accomplish in four to six weeks, particularly given the time it takes to become oriented to the site and organization. Be sure to factor in the availability of mentorship and staff, especially considering holidays or other local scheduling considerations.

Regardless of the form of the program, elements to seek in a sound international rotation include a sustained relationship between the home organization or participants and the host organization. In the case of an individual project, working on a site where you have long-term collaboration is more likely to fulfill your objectives and the site's needs. In the case of organizations, look for continuous communication to assess and respond to local priorities as indicators of sound relationships. Previous participants will be an excellent source of information on how well the program is able to integrate you within the health facility or organization. As Dr. Wilfrido Torres says regarding Child Family Health International

(CFHI), among the hallmarks of a good program are, "Acceptable remuneration [for mentors], permanent communication that overcomes the language barrier, donation of materials that strengthen the local affiliated clinics, help with local initiatives, the link with the Teaching and Learning that we develop with the students, help with local training, and the opportunity for professional development." Strong communication and commitment to local priorities provide the groundwork for successful individual rotations.

Mentorship and Supervision: No matter your level of experience, you are sure to encounter unfamiliar situations, cultural aspects, and health concerns, for which you will need local guidance. Most trainees who participate in international rotations find significant worth in good local support, some supervision, and a decent amount of mentorship. The amount and quality of mentorship may reflect the commitment of the home institution to indentifying and supporting host mentors who have the time and inclination to work with visiting students. Some issues to consider include:

- Does the rotation site provide mentors? How much experience do they have working with trainees?
- Will the mentor be able to commit to assisting you during your rotation? It may be beneficial to develop specific expectations about time with a mentor, particularly based on the experience of other students or residents at a site. How often do you anticipate checking in with a mentor? Do you anticipate working closely with him or her?
- Will the mentor be away from the host site for any part of your stay? If so, are there ways to identify other mentors to work with?
- Is it possible to be in contact prior to departure to develop projects and to learn about site and community before you leave?
- What other support may be available from the site, such as a visitor liaison to assist with logistics?

Infrastructure and Logistics – Housing:
- Is there a safe place where you can be housed near the site?
- If housing is provided, is it a dorm room, home-stay, or separate residence? Will you be living with other visiting students and residents or will you be living alone?
- How much does it cost? Consider rent as well as transit and food expenses in determining if you can afford this accommodation. In urban areas, less expensive housing may be located in areas where there is limited safe public transport and a taxi or driver is required, particularly at night.

- Will you be able to walk, take safe public transport, or need to take private transport (e.g. hire taxis or a driver) to travel between your housing and the rotation site?
- Is your housing safe enough for you? Determine what safety measures are in place for your own security and to protect your valuables, including security guards, safe boxes, locks, etc.
- Will you be able to cook on site? If so, is there an accessible food market? Will your meals be prepared for you? Will you need to eat out? Can you afford this?
- Will your housing have electricity, running water, flushing toilets (versus out-houses or latrines), a telephone line, access to shops and eateries, etc.?
- With regard to rent, be sure to clarify in advance the amount, due date, where rent is paid, and how to pay rent (cash, check, etc.) and pay it on time and in full. Programs usually do not have funds to cover missed payments by visitors.

Cost:
- What does the program provide for you? For example, the cost of a language program may include a home-stay, some meals, day-long classes, and some trips.
- How much can you afford to pay? Will you be able to afford the program you're interested in? Factor in travel (both internationally and in-country,) visa, program, accommodations, meals, vaccinations, and supply costs.
- Are scholarships or fellowships available to help cover the cost? The American Medical Student Association's (AMSA's) website lists some of the available scholarships and fellowships: http://www.amsa.org/AMSA/Homepage/About/Committees/Global/FundingYourTrip.aspx

Part 2 – Prepping for your rotation

AMSA's website has a "Checklist for Going Abroad" that you can download: http://www.amsa.org/AMSA/Libraries/Committee_Docs/abroad_checklist.sflb.ashx. Your institution or program may also provide preparation or orientation materials specific to the site.

A. Language

You will need to communicate, whether or not you know the language of the place that you are going. Dr. Daniel Kwaro, formerly the Program Systems Coordinator for the FACES program in Kenya (which hosts many visiting students, residents and researchers), says, "However good or smart

111

you are, if you're not a people person, don't go." You will be relying on people at your site to help you survive while you are there, and they are relying on you to make a positive contribution, so it is important that you are able to communicate with them. It's fine not to be fluent or perfect or even verbal; the most important thing is that you are respectful and you earnestly try to communicate.

Learn common respectful greetings and gratitude in the native language before you go. Ideally, if you don't already speak the native language, find a tutor or a class through which you can learn basic conversational language and a few key medical terms if you will be working with patients (e.g. hurt, pain, sick, where, when, head, lung, stomach, etc.). You can fill in more medical terminology later. Look for a portable dictionary or phrasebook that you can refer to and learn from while you are in the host community.

Cultural competency can be critical to success in a new community. It can be very helpful to learn cultural nuances and to consider the appropriateness of certain terminology and expressions. For example, many cultures do not use sarcasm as a way to communicate (as is used in North America and Europe). Sarcastic remarks can be confusing and condescending in such cultures. Remember that even English-speaking countries will use language differently. Slang will be especially different. For example, if you are from the US and go to a place that uses British English, people there will say "trousers" instead of "pants" or "petrol" instead of "gas." Accents and patterns of speech will also differ. As Dr. S.M. Dabak and Dr. S.S. Dabak of the CFHI Program in Pune, India note, students and residents "should talk slowly and clearly with doctors, nurses, and so on. They should make sure that the person with whom they are talking has understood what they have spoken."

Be aware of different standards of beauty and age. For example, in some cultures, older age is associated with wisdom and respect; physical size and weight may be linked to wealth or beauty. Try to take comments on appearance and age in context.

B. Place

Prepare as much as possible before you arrive. Learn about the country and area where you will work, including the clinical environment and the diagnostic and treatment options available. The World Health Organization (WHO) website includes many free, up-to-date, downloadable resources, including region-specific epidemiology and health care guidelines. Try to learn about common illnesses for that area, particularly tropical diseases with which you are not familiar. For instance, a large number of fresh water lakes and rivers in Africa contain schistosomiasis parasites. Learn about schistosomiasis before traveling so you can make an informed decision about your level of exposure. This information is especially important given that all cultures have their own conceptions and beliefs about health and illness. Traveling residents may be forced to choose between following medical knowledge and the community belief about risk and exposure while traveling. Look for country-specific guidelines if you have access to them. For example, many countries have their own guidelines on how to treat tuberculosis, malaria, and HIV.

Get in touch with other students, residents or researchers who have previously worked at your proposed site. Many academic institutions provide databases of international projects which can help you identify people with experience at or near your project site; administrative staff within the international or global health office can also be an excellent source of information. Preparation about the host location will help visiting residents acclimate faster once they are in the community.

C. Communication

Cell phones:
- If you have a cell phone that is compatible with international SIM cards (e.g. quad-band), call your cell phone company and request the SIM card unlock code and instructions. If you can unlock your phone or if it is already unlocked, you can purchase a SIM card at your international site when you arrive. When you have unlocked your phone and inserted the international-site SIM card, voila! You now have a local cell phone number.
- Learn about local cell phone charges. Pre-paid credits that you add to your SIM card are a common method of payment.
- SMS (text messages) are often much cheaper than talking on the phone, so you may find texting a more convenient and affordable alternative.
- In some regions, you will be charged for making calls, but it is free to receive calls. Especially with host community contacts, co-workers and friends, keep in mind that you may have cell phone credit while others may not.
- "Flashes" (when someone calls your phone and then hangs up after it rings) are part of some cultures, and are a way of saying, "Please call me." People sometimes don't have enough credit on their phones to make a call but need to get in touch with you, so they are asking you to call them back.

Internet:
- Many travelers find slow or unreliable internet connections to be very frustrating. Be aware in advance that you will probably not have the internet speed and reliability you are used to and consider this in your planning (i.e. Is it the best time to submit residency applications while working in Africa?)

- In some regions, it is most reliable to use your cell phone as a modem or to get a SIM-card modem. This type of modem set-up uses the telephone network to access the internet, which is often more reliable than the satellite internet connection in some areas. Prior to your rotation, it might be useful to check if you can use your phone as a modem and find out how to do it. You will likely need to use region-specific software when you buy a new SIM card in the host country.
- Learn how to use Skype (www.skype.com) or Google Chat. These programs allow you to contact people at home cheaply and reliably.

D. Packing

- Pack light! Prior to leaving, lay out everything that you are thinking of taking with you. Some experienced travelers would advise to halve that quantity and bring twice the amount of money with you. If you're not sure whether you need something, you probably don't need it. Many places will not accept credit cards for purchases. However, ATMs and banks in urban areas generally accept debit cards for cash withdrawal. It is very important to notify your bank prior to your departure so that international transactions are not blocked. Investigate transaction fees and obtain an international contact number to reach the bank in case of emergency.
- Check out the "Ultimate Trip Prep and Packing List." [www.resister.info/trip-pack-list.pdf] Review it at least three months before you leave so you can get your vaccines, passport, visas, and supplies in order.
- Make copies of your essential documents – passport, visa, health insurance card, airplane tickets if applicable – and leave them with an emergency contact. Your institution may also request a copy in case of emergencies, and should at least be able to reach your emergency contact. It may be useful to have a scanned copy of these documents accessible on your email as well.
- Put your most important items (passport, large bills, insurance and health information) in a slim waist belt that you can wear under your clothes.
- Bring appropriate clothing for the site. Dress codes may not be the same at health clinics or hospitals as they are in the U.S. For instance, students and residents are not generally permitted to wear scrubs in hospitals in Mexico. Many health facilities expect business or business casual attire from their staff; be respectful in following these routines. It is important to remember that even though the conditions in a host community may be unfamiliar or

even initially uncomfortable, your clothing and appearance are statement to community members about you and your institution.

- Leave space in your luggage for gifts and purchases for when you are abroad.
- Specific items that can help with global health rotations
    - Contact the program and the site to see if there are certain things they want you to bring before packing, such as medical supplies and donated items. Students and residents who have previously rotated at the site may also have recommendations. You may also want to check if there are specific teaching sessions that would be useful to prepare, so that you can do research or gather useful material in advance.
    - If you are rotating in a location with limited access to hand washing, bring hand sanitizer to use and a large quantity to leave with clinical staff.
    - Bring the medical equipment that you will need while at your site.
    - Consider bringing extra stethoscopes, extra copies of pocket reference books and reference CDs (e.g., UpToDate©, collections of relevant articles as PDF) to leave with host site clinical staff.
    - Consider fun gifts to leave with all staff and hosts (regional gifts, chocolates, candies, stickers for kids, etc.) It may be important to ask host site staff, especially in a clinical setting, if you can distribute such gifts or if they would like to distribute them.
    - Postcards or pictures from your home area or institution can be a nice way to share where you are from with hosts and friends.
    - Bring personal items that you may not be able to buy in the host community (e.g., medications [malaria prophylaxis, antibiotics, antidiarrheals, previously prescribed medications], tampons, condoms, lube, hand sanitizer, etc.)
    - A few doses of low-dose melatonin can sometimes help with jet lag and adjustment to radically different time zones.
    - Bring ear plugs and something to cover your eyes with (bandana, eye mask) so you can sleep despite time and noise changes.

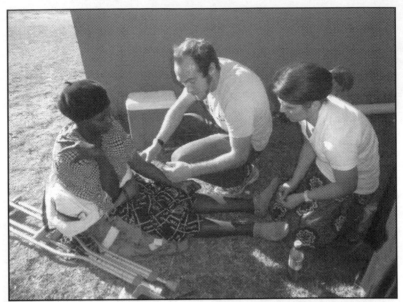

Stephen Donnelly and Megan Little, first year medical students at Wright State University, explain the importance of regular HIV testing to a female patient in Swaziland, during their summer elective as part of the school's Global Health Initiative. (Photo credit: Alicia Boyd)

During the Rotation

Part 1 – Landing: getting your bearings when you first arrive

A. Observe and absorb your new setting

If this is your first time at the site, spend at least a few days after you arrive to soak up the sights, sounds, culture and language of your new surroundings. Meet locals and do what they do. Remember that you are a guest: respect local customs and boundaries and go where you are welcome. Continue to do this during your free time: make friends with local co-workers and take them up on their offers to hang out and show you around. It is important that you understand that you are entering a different community and that you learn from it and adapt to it as best you can. Only then can you make a positive contribution.

Expatriates often make their own enclaves and exclusive communities. Remember that old saying, 'When in Rome, do as the Romans do.' Try to break out of ex-pat enclaves, learn a bit of the local language, and try to be open and make friends with local folks. You can start by getting to know the people with whom you are working in clinics or

116

research sites. If you invite someone to join you for a meal, to go out, etc, keep in mind that they might assume you are paying. If that is not your intention then clarify early. At least once, put away your tour book, phone and camera, and go out and enjoy a walk.

B. Psychological preparation

Have large eyes, large ears, and a small mouth. The most important piece of advice we can give you is to keep an open mind. You may feel overwhelmed by the amount of poverty you see. You may feel alienated by being obviously an outsider. You may get followed by curious children or harassed by young men trying to make extra cash. You may be called names that you consider rude or inappropriate. Be ready to accept the situation as it is. It may not be out of disrespect. Many problems that you see are due to problems in the system, circumstances and larger society, not due to individual decisions. As Dr. Torres suggests, keep in mind that visitors "are not capable of saving the world; generally the locations have their potential and mechanisms that allow them to survive. Though we recognize that there are serious health problems, generally the solution is not held by a foreigner, but is a conjunction of local, participatory actions." Bear in mind that you are there primarily to learn, to provide short-term support for clinical care, and to meet and work with your local colleagues, not to pass judgment or to implement systemic change.

Learn to empathize with local providers' and staff situations. Some may work evening and weekend jobs to make extra money as they may not earn adequate pay from public clinic jobs . You may see providers and staff leave long queues of patients waiting to work at their other jobs. Rather than get upset or angry, reflect on the balance of forces in this situation – you may be able to help care for some of these patients.

Be prepared to feel upset and cry. Depending on the location and clinical nature of your site, you may see death at your clinical site, much of which you may consider to be preventable. Keep in mind that there are a multitude of cultural nuances and practices when it comes to encountering death. Local providers may not demonstrate the same level of distress because they have experienced it many times before and understand the limitations of their setting. You may also feel incredibly lonely at times while you are away from your friends and family at home. Finally, remember that all places have crime. Try not to allow small negative incidents to taint your full experience.

Part 2 – Making the most of your experience

A. Health, Safety, Comfort and Hygiene
- Make sure to understand how to access your international health insurance while you are abroad. Carry that information and a

photocopy of your passport with you at all times (e.g. in your waist pouch).

- Leave a copy of your passport, travel insurance and emergency contact details with a responsible person at the rotation site and at home.
- Have contact numbers for at least two local people who can assist you in case of emergency.
- Identify the nearest quality health care provider (e.g. international or private-pay health centers and hospitals) and keep that contact information with your health insurance information. When you seek medical care from a provider, private hospitals often provide better quality care than public facilities for those who can pay.
- Keep in mind that in many regions, you can get medications from private "chemists" or "pharmacists" on the street. Many of these outlets do not undergo quality-control; oftentimes, it is safer to obtain medications from government-run or public hospitals that are quality controlled.
- Many people feel uninhibited while traveling or more open to new experiences. Remember to continue to use your good judgment and be aware of situations when your judgment may be impaired, such as after alcohol intake.
- Use alcohol in moderation and be wary of local brews.
- Regardless of what any local may tell you, buying, selling, or using illegal drugs while traveling is extremely dangerous. DO NOT expect the U.S. State Department to provide anything but minimal support if you are caught breaking local laws. It is your responsibility to know and follow the laws.
- Meeting new people is part of the fun and one of the best parts of the experience. However, entering into personal relationships, including intimate ones, comes with additional risks and complications. Cultural expectations and boundaries may be very different than yours. Also, consider the personal risks that a local may face by being in a relationship with you. Unprotected sex is never a good idea, and is dangerous in many settings.
- Cover your body! Dress as conservatively as conservative locals. Dress in layers.
- Wear comfortable shoes, sunscreen or a cover-up, and a smile.
- Always carry toilet paper and hand sanitizer.
- After all that.... you will have a great experience. Remember: "don't be so cautious that you miss the magic."[3]

---

[3] Nicolas Kristof, New York Times, 5/31/09.

B. Transportation

- Learn how to use the local public transportation system. The biggest public buses are often the safest routes of travel.
- Avoid biking in a city without bike lanes or that is not bike-friendly.
- Find out from community members where the safest walking routes are. Try to avoid walking alone in the dark.
- Maintain safe following distances when walking or biking.
- In general, avoid traveling at night. It is more dangerous for many reasons including poor lighting, increased numbers of drunk drivers, and higher risk of theft or mugging.
- Ask site staff for phone numbers of reliable taxi drivers.
- Notify a local point-person that you trust (home-stay family, supervisor, co-worker, or friend) of any trips you are taking so they know where you are in case of an emergency. You may be involved in an accident and need local contacts to help you to find the care you need.
- Use a seat belt whenever possible, even if nobody else is. This cannot be emphasized enough!

C. Food and Eating

- Choose cooked and still-hot foods (i.e. recently cooked foods, not food that's been sitting around). Vegetarians: beware of salads.
- Always bring hand sanitizer and use it. Your GI tract may not be accustomed to the local food and microorganisms.
- Boil water to a vigorous boil for at least one minute to kill pathogenic microorganisms and make drinking water. Bring a reusable and durable water bottle to refill rather than purchasing and wasting disposable water bottles while you're there. Avoid ice.
- Explore local markets and learn how to make local foods, especially if you have access to a kitchen.
- If you go to someone's house for a meal, tell them in advance if you have food allergies or restrictions. It's better to warn them ahead of time than to suffer through a meal you cannot eat. (Your host will probably be more amused than think that you are rude or picky.)
- Look for a place to eat before you are starving: you might be waiting for much longer than you anticipated for the food! Keep in mind that if a restaurant is empty, there is often a good reason for that.
- Leaving a tip may not be customary; as your hosts about standard expectations in the area.
- If you are sharing kitchen and cooking space with others, be sensitive to the expectations about sharing food and space. For

example, rather than labeling each food item with your name or "don't touch!", consider keeping food that you do not want to share in your own room.

D. Impact and Contributions

- Be aware of your impact on individuals and programs. Most people will go out of their way to be hospitable and accommodate you. Hosts may even do this at the expense of themselves, patients, and limited resources. Think about the impact to others before you ask for something.
- Remember you are a representative for your home institution and for your home country. Act in a way that reflects well on both.
- You will undoubtedly want to contribute to the site you are working in either clinically, via research, or through donations. Make your contributions thoughtful and useful in the local context. Teaching and sharing of knowledge and experiences is an excellent way in which we can all contribute. (See tips on "Teaching in International Settings" below).

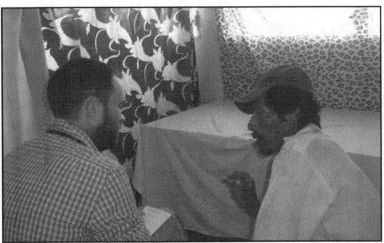

Matthew Kutcher, MD and a patient from the community of Campo Uno, RAAN, Nicaragua during a clinic visit. (Photo credit: Susan Hadley.)

E. Research

It's important to be flexible and open to your site's needs and priorities. Researchers often conceptualize projects in their home country, and then search for a developing country site in which they can conduct the study.

Different levels of collaboration between "global north and south" country[4] institutions will occur during conceptualization, planning, and implementation, but these projects are often dominated by the "north" country's input. Although the study topic may be important to the home researcher, be aware that it may not match the priority questions faced by clinicians and program planners at the host or rotation site.

Research projects should be focused on areas the local program feels are important and with as much input and collaboration as possible by local communities and health professionals. If you are interested in implementing your own research project, it will be much more feasible to do so working with local collaborators and responding to the needs that they identify. Remember that tasks will take you *at least* twice as long to do as you expect and plan accordingly. For a short rotation, contributing to an existing research project is likely to be more worthwhile than attempting to initiate and complete a new project of your own. It is often very difficult to complete an overly ambitious research project in four to six weeks at an unfamiliar site with new colleagues and co-workers.

Keep in mind that any research intended for publication requires multiple levels of authorization, including institutional review board clearance at both your home institution and a local institution, a process that can require six months or more to navigate. Implementing a research protocol also frequently requires organizational approval from local institutions, whether a ministry of health or an academic institution. It is essential to learn about the organizational structure of your project site and any required approvals.

It is also beneficial to identify the key stakeholders within and beyond the health facility beforehand, with assistance from your local mentor or contacts. Needs assessment and key stakeholder interviews may be arranged more effectively through your local mentor. Just as at an academic institution in the U.S., it can take time to coordinate meetings. If possible, you should introduce your research project to all staff at the site when you arrive, and without fail, you should disseminate preliminary and final results back to the staff.

Other best practices include:

- Adapt and modify protocols once you have arrived and learned about the existing systems that you will use. Try to figure out a way to fit your data collection and research into the local system with minimal disruption, rather than asking clinical staff to accommodate to your schedule and structure.
- Try not to take resources away from patient care. Be aware that clinicians may be more interested and occupied by providing patient care than performing research.

---

[4] The "global north and south" refers to countries in the Northern Hemisphere and the Southern Hemisphere with regard to economic and technological resources; a more recent alternative to describe "developed" and "developing countries."

- Learn to push gently. If you are relying on local staff to do some of the work, understand that they have their own responsibilities and competing priorities. Learn to remind them diplomatically of their role in your project and help them set aside resources and time to do so. For example, if you are also a clinician, help see some of their patients or get other clinical work done so that you help free up their time.
- While you are on site and conducting your study, take the time to find out what other questions need to be answered as a priority for the site so you can bring those ideas back to your institution for future projects.
- Give a presentation on your preliminary findings before you leave to share your work with the local staff. Frequently, local staff who have participated in your research do not get to read or hear about the final research results and findings.
- Remember, small accomplishments are important.

F. Clinical Work

Clinical work in resource-limited settings has many constraints that you can't foresee and control, so it is important to be flexible, patient, diligent and persistent. You can't do everything for everyone. Celebrate the small accomplishments.

- Identify a supervisor as early as possible. Make every effort to meet with that person during your first few days of the rotation (preferably schedule the appointment in advance) to discuss expectations, roles as a clinician, researcher or teacher, objectives, and other potential projects that may be helpful. Schedule a brief mid-rotation meeting to discuss how things are going – this may not seem important for a four-week rotation, but it is helpful for the visiting resident and the host site. Schedule an end-of-rotation meeting for evaluation of your work, of the elective site, and of your supervisor. Even if there is not a system in place for formal evaluation, make an effort to go through this process as it benefits all parties.
- Keep your eyes open for unexpected ways to be helpful. Beyond clinical work, there may be quality improvement projects you can work on, systems issues to help solve, grant writing for projects, CME sessions, literature reviews, or other projects. Dr. German Tenorio of CFHI Oaxaca suggests, "that the resident conducts him or herself in a broader environment than the doctor-patient relationship, for instance teaching, media and communication, and overall health systems."
- Pick one (just one!) clinical area to focus on while you are there for teaching and clinical skills improvement. It's best to

- communicate with local staff before or when you arrive to choose the topic. Some programs may maintain lists of useful teaching sessions; prior residents may also have suggestions.
- Knowledge sharing is a two-way process, be open to teaching by peers, mentors and co-workers, and your teaching will be better received.
- If you can communicate about it before you arrive, prepare images or slides, articles and teaching materials to bring with you. Remember that you have limited time there, so be realistic. Learn to pick the lowest hanging fruit.
- Consider how you can contribute beyond the clinical personnel; for instance, refresher training sessions on basic skills for paramedical personnel may be extremely useful. Remember to make these sessions relevant to the health concerns and resources specific to the site.
- Plan for and make a presentation, teaching session or CME on a topic that matches local interests (which ideally coordinates with the topic you've chosen above). See more details in the section below on teaching.
- Acknowledge your level of expertise. Don't let staff or patient pressure push you to go beyond your competence. Staff and patients will often have an unrealistic expectation of your abilities simply because you come from a highly resourced country.
- You may see many things that are done differently than in your past experience. You may have a lot of ideas on improvements that can be made. Make notes of these and find the appropriate people with whom to discuss them (usually the coordinators/directors or appropriate department managers) during a meeting scheduled for that purpose. Do not constantly make suggestions on how people can improve what they are doing, particularly to those who do not make program planning decisions.
- Many countries have fairly clear national guidelines for diagnosis and treatment of malaria, TB, and HIV. You can find many of them on the WHO website and the country's national public health website. It is important to follow and promote the guidelines when possible, to maintain consistency for clinical staff and also because of implications for supply management, reporting, and planning, all of which are generally designed around the guidelines.
- Hone your skills in international diplomacy. If you find that a clinician is not following guidelines, present the protocol as an alternative option. For example, you can say, "Do you think that this antibiotic might be better for gram-positives? Shall we look it up together in the *Sanford Guide*?" If the clinician does not have a *Sanford Guide to Antimicrobial Therapy* and you've brought extras, then plan to leave a copy with them.

- When you are seeing patients, learn to triage quickly. Help other staff do the same. You can refer to the WHO Integrated Management of Adolescent and Adult Illness (IMAI) or Integrated Management of Childhood Illness (IMCI) guidelines. Recognize clinical limitations early: when you don't know or are not sure what to do, refer to others who are better trained or are in a higher-intensity hospital setting with better resources. No one individual can know everything or can do everything. Practice and model recognition of limits and work as a conscientious team member in order to provide patients with the appropriate level of care.
- Clinical staff and non-physicians in resource-limited settings are often trained algorithmically, so if there is time, demonstrate and teach how to think through a differential diagnosis.
- Appreciate the time constraints of staff and work with the situation. For example, if your mentoring and teaching is slowing down the flow of patients and/or not allowing clinicians to see patients (who have often waited since dawn!), ask the clinicians what they think would be the best use of their time. Consider spending a limited part of the day teaching and then the rest of the day helping them see patients efficiently.
- Model resource-appropriate clinical behaviors and skills. For example, most clinicians in resource-limited settings don't have updated Epocrates© on PDAs. Dr. Jeremy Penner, Associate Director, Division of Global Health, Department of Family Practice, at the University of British Columbia, says, "When I was doing a residency elective in Haiti, I spent time working with a nurse who had been there for around 10 years, but often traveled back to the US. I asked why she didn't use a PDA as a quick reference for drug dosages, diagnostic reference, etc. She explained that although it would be convenient for her, it does not model a behavior that the other staff could use. We want to encourage people to use reference material or consult when they don't know something (rather than just guess, which happens too often), but using a technology which most of the health workers do not have access to does not help. Using handbooks such as Sanford guides and Pharmacopeias, or free internet resources (if at a site with internet access) such as MD Consult, allows you to model a behavior that is accessible. Particularly if you can bring extra copies to leave behind."
- Hand in a formal appraisal of the site and of your supervisor BEFORE you leave the site. If there is no structure or format for this, then use one from your home institution of develop your own. Keep a copy for future reference.
- Fulfill your time commitment and pre-arranged responsibilities to the site, and take the site schedule seriously. Arrive on time, avoid

long lunches, short afternoons, or long weekends. Schedule holiday and travel time before or after the rotation.

G. Communication in Clinical Settings
Remember: Have large eyes, large ears, and a small mouth.

- Before you speak, pause, take a breath and think before you open your mouth. As Dr. German Tenorio of CFHI Mexico says, "A student who asks questions with courtesy, who knows to wait for the response, who isn't bothered if they are ignored at the time, is a student who will find many answers."
- When talking to a clinician or staff person about something to improve upon, use a feedback sandwich: praise / feedback / praise. For example, "You are working hard and doing a great job seeing so many patients a day. I've noticed that perhaps we can work on improving this protocol so that we can provide even better care for our patients. I can see that you have the smarts, dedication and persistence to do this well."

H. Teaching
Host programs are often very eager for visitors to participate in knowledge exchange in the form of one-on-one mentoring, small group activities like journal clubs or case discussions, or large group presentations. Remember that you will have much more to learn in this setting than to teach, and take this opportunity to learn about local issues and to share some of your expertise. If you are able to provide mentoring about a topic or are interested in being mentored in a specific area, it may be helpful to establish specific learning objectives prior to your rotation.

The following are a few tips for presentations:

Choosing a Topic:
- During your first week on-site, you can take an informal poll among the clinical staff on topics they would like to discuss. It is often interesting to present both the local as well as the "developed country" way of approaching and managing a disease, even if the local staff doesn't have access to the same diagnostics and treatments. Present the differences rationally so that the staff understands world-wide practices in a non-judgmental way.
- Consider your comfort level with the topic
- Note that presentations done in US often lack relevance and applicability. It's fine to include what happens in resource-rich countries but also very important to present what can be done locally.
- Be prepared to adjust pre-fabricated presentations considerably

125

Format:
- Consider what is appropriate given the audience and setting (Journal club, skills demonstration, clinical practice, knowledge review, introducing new medical advances)

Setting:
- Know the resources available locally, local knowledge and cultural implications.
- Have a host co-worker review your presentation.
- Don't count on being able to give a computer-generated (e.g. PowerPoint) presentation. Other formats may better fit your audience (small group, chalk board, flip chart, interactive). If you decide to use a computer presentation, always have a back-up plan in case of a power blackout or equipment malfunction.

Afterwards: following-up and reflecting

Be careful about making commitments that require follow-up upon return home. We have the best intentions when on site, but upon returning to school or residency we have to make that learning environment our priority and often cannot fulfill commitments made in our rotation site. As a simple example, many people take pictures but do not even send them back to the staff.

Reflect on the sustainability of your actions. Foreign presence and funding will never be more than a temporary solution. NGO money tends to patch up problems rather than build full systematic responses. You may not be able to fix this, but if you are mindful, you can help the staff become more skillful and self-sustaining. Realize the impact of your work on the entire community.

Studies show that students who participate in global health rotations are more likely to choose career paths in global health or working with the underserved and often experience a change in approach to medicine upon their return, such as considering how many lab tests are truly required. While you will have some reverse culture shock upon return, try to maintain and share some of the things you learned during your travels and apply them to the work you continue to do at home. If you would be willing to discuss your experience with future residents, it may be helpful to notify a program coordinator or residency director and give contact information. Alternatively, writing a short summary of your impressions of the site and valuable information you wish you had known prior to your rotation is extremely helpful for future students and residents. Whether or not you return to a particular site or pursue international work in the future, the impact of your global health rotation can endure well beyond the experience itself.

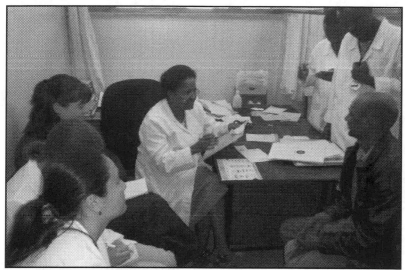

Fourth year medical students from the Medical School for International Health in Beer Sheva, Israel visit a Dermatology clinic in Addis Ababa, Ethiopia as part of a 7 week international medicine clerkship. (Photo credit: Jonathan Mendelsohn.)

Kelly Anderson and Melanie Anspacher

> *One's mind, once stretched by a new idea never regains its original dimensions.*
> Oliver Wendell Holmes

The power of mentorship cannot be underestimated. After residency, individuals emerge from years of rigorous medical training to take on the role of a physician. Residency is a period of socialization in which physicians develop an understanding of the responsibilities, boundaries and opportunities involved in providing health care. It is critical to have guidance through this formative period. The right mentor, at the right time, can provide insight, inspire, and encourage a resident as a physician and as a person. Especially in the expanding discipline of global health, a seasoned mentor can shed light on experiences, provide a sounding board, and guide us in academic and educational pursuits. A mentor can clarify the current problem, but, perhaps more importantly, the right mentor can encourage us to think broadly about what else is possible. Mentorship can assist young leaders to thoughtfully develop their goals and aspirations. Even a small act of encouragement on the part of a mentor can make a life-changing difference for a resident on the cusp of transformation.

The following chapter will review recent mentorship literature and apply it to global health training to address the definition of mentorship, qualities of effective mentees and mentors, support for mentors, and initiation, structure and evaluation of mentorship. It will also provide specific considerations for mentors regarding global health training opportunities.

Definition of Mentorship

A mentor has been described as an influential and trusted counselor, guide, teacher, coach or supporter. By employing expertise or experience in a shared interest, a mentor contributes to the development of a mentee in personal and professional capacities. According to *Berk et al.*, the academic mentoring relationship:

> *may vary along a continuum from informal/short term to formal/long term in which faculty with useful experience, knowledge skills and/or wisdom offers advice, information, guidance, support or opportunity to another faculty member or student for that individual's professional development.*[1]

It has been described that a mentor's hindsight can become the mentee's foresight. "Functional mentoring," in which the relationship centers on the project at hand, can provide specific guidance.[2] This may be a particularly pertinent definition when applied to global health electives for students and residents.

Who Can Be a Global Health Faculty Mentor?

Global health is an interdisciplinary field that generally defies a specific unifying definition, despite rigorous attempts.[3] Given that the field is interdisciplinary and continually evolving, there is a wide scope for potential global health mentors. The Global Health Mentorship Project (http://ghmp.cfms.org) is a Canadian initiative that links undergraduate medical students with mentors in global health. It attracts mentors from the fields of medicine, nursing, paramedics, non-profit management, non-governmental organizations and health policy. In yearly evaluations of this project, the majority of mentees find this experience to be useful, and the utility does not correlate with having a physician as a mentor. When physicians are selected for global health mentors, community-oriented physicians are often the first to be considered. However, practitioners from many fields may provide practical mentorship for an open-minded resident interested in global health. For example, a resident approaching an upcoming domestic or international medical elective may find the best fit with an international development expert, or social worker familiar with the community of interest.

In the case of physician-mentors, there is no definitive type or level of experience in global health to ensure success. The experience level of a physician mentor may vary from recent residency graduates with global health experience, to senior physicians committed to globally focused research or long-term clinical work. Faculty at different stages in their career may be able to serve in different yet equally valuable mentoring roles.[4] Early career physicians may be better able to relate to the current trainees, and may be more familiar with residency program requirements and challenges to pursuing global health experiences. Many young physicians have completed global health electives or short-term work in low-resource settings. Having often forged their own path in global health, such early career mentors may be very eager to share their experience with others. Faculty who are in the middle to late career stages may have more expertise to share, more established reputations, more contacts in the field, and more institutional influence; however, they may have less time to dedicate to mentorship. The former may be better suited to serve as a mentor for residents preparing for their global health electives or projects, while the latter may be better suited to serving as career or curriculum advisors. It may be useful for a resident to have two or more mentors that are at different stages of their careers. Residents may benefit from "layering" their mentors – discussing the details of a global health elective with a mentor who recently finished training, while seeking broader professional guidance from more experienced advisors.

As in the Global Health Mentorship Project, programs with a limited number of institutional global health mentors may recruit local and international affiliates and extramural advisors. Resources include special interest sections and groups of professional societies, young physician networks, public health schools, non-governmental and community-based organizations. Once identified, physicians, allied health professionals and community development workers may welcome the opportunity to share their expertise as global health mentors with physicians currently in training.

Cultivating Effective Mentors

Although little has been established on the ideal qualities of a global health faculty mentor, there is a wealth of literature on attributes of effective mentors in medical education. *Jackson et al.* identified the central importance of a mentor's knowledge of the mentee, in order to envision the mentee's possibilities.[5] Prerequisite qualities for a mentor include dedication to both the idea of mentorship and the mentee, and adequate time to engage in the relationship. Another quality identified by *Jackson et al.* is a willingness to support and enable the mentee. In the global health context, a mentor might assist in development of contacts, identification of critical organizations and connection to major partners in the sector of interest.

Sambunjak et al. synthesized six studies reporting the desired characteristics of a mentor into three categories, which relate to the mentor's personality, interpersonal abilities and professional status.[6] Overall, the study concluded that successful mentors should be sincere and honest, listen actively and try to gauge the needs of the mentee, create a safe space for expression of thought and emotion, and facilitate goal setting and self-reflection. The study also noted the importance of a mentor's established reputation in his or her sector. Similarly to *Jackson et al*, the study found that mentors should enhance mentees' visibility and connections within the sector of interest and, "to protect them from adverse influences and harsh interactions."

Some additional qualities of an effective mentor may include:

- clear and effective communication
- establishment of trust
- displays of investment and motivation
- commitment to mentoring as part of his or her professional role

- willingness to share personal experiences
- interest in the goals and aspirations of a mentee
- encouragement of independent decision-making

An effective mentor will be a role model, while also guiding the mentee to pursue his or her own interests and providing constructive feedback. Perhaps most importantly, a mentor will be accountable to the structure set out in the mentorship based on shared expectations, whether informal or formal. A mentor must hold the mentee accountable to shared agreements.

Cultivating Effective Mentees

For mentorship to be successful, the mentee must take responsibility and initiative to create and sustain the partnership. Many studies emphasize the importance of a mentee's active management of the mentoring relationship.[2,6,7,8,9] Effective mentorship truly begins when a mentee possesses the right degree of interest, motivation and skills to initiate, cultivate and facilitate a relationship with a mentor. This mentee leadership has been described as sitting in the "driver's seat."[8] In their systematic review, *Sambunjak et al.* explored and summarized the development, perceptions and experiences of mentoring relationships in academic medicine. They noted that passion to succeed, pro-activity, willingness to learn are critical attributes in an effective mentee. They also suggested that mentees should prepare for meetings with their mentors, provide a suggested outline for each discussion, and complete assigned tasks. Mentees should also respond honestly to feedback and accept suggestions constructively. Mentees should regularly self-reflect and bring these insights to the mentorship discussion, so the mentor can provide input. The authors emphasized that effective mentorship requires courage on behalf of the mentee.

A critical and often unexplored level of this discussion is how mentees can actively seek out effective, informal mentorship. This is particularly relevant to global health mentorship as mentees may have difficulty locating appropriate mentors in their home institutions. Persistence is also often required in finding a mentor. In order to further investigate mentoring, and to examine the "mystery" of effective mentorship alliances, *Jackson et al.* conducted individual telephone interviews of 16 young faculty members about seeking mentorship.[5] One interviewee suggested, "Advice that I do give… is to go set up a half hour appointment with everyone in your department. Just go sit and talk with them and that way you start to find out who would be the natural mentors." Another participant added, "I would persevere and if you don't find someone who's suitable in your department or in your institution, then think of people beyond. But I think you have to go get it set up yourself. People

aren't just going to fall into your lap and say, 'I want to be your mentor.'"
The study noted that mentees may find that several people, rather than one individual, better provide comprehensive mentorship.

This is not to diminish the role of a mentor in cultivating the relationship, but to encourage residency programs to train residents to be mentees. This type of training may increase successful location of mentors and the success of mentoring relationships. Indeed, formal mentorship programs do not guarantee "the right chemistry" between mentors and mentees, but innovative and initiative-taking residents often find the right fit through an informal mentor search.[5] To help interested residents form mentorships in global health, a broad search – in several disciplines or across teaching centers – may be useful. As will be elaborated later on, global health mentors can come from multiple fields and will not necessarily be found exclusively within the faculty base at their institutions. It may also be useful in addition to a formal mentorship program, to bring interested residents and potential mentors together, both socially and professionally, in a systematic way early in the residency program. This can facilitate connections between keen, passionate and motivated residents who and potential like-minded mentors early on.

Support for Mentors

Cultivating effective global health mentors requires support for mentors. Institutions which undertake formal or informal mentorship in global health should consider how to support mentorship as part of the culture of their organization. In a recent review of the literature, five articles discussed the need for improved institutional support and recognition of mentors. *Rammani et al.* conducted a series of workshops with medical faculty to identify key elements of training in mentorship programs.[10] These workshops identified focus areas of interpersonal boundaries, forums to discuss uncertainties and problems, evaluation strategies, protected time, reward systems and recognition. In their systematic literature review, *Sambunjak et al.* cite several structural barriers to effective mentorship including lack of time, lack of energy due to overwhelming logistical and tactical problems, lack of recognition and incentive for mentors and a limited pool of available mentors. They propose incentives of protected time, formal evaluations and awards. In their article, *Thorndyke et al.* describe the effective mentor rewards initiative at the Penn State College Junior Faculty Development Program. This mentorship program lasts one year and relies on voluntary mentors who are formally recognized and inducted into the "mentorship academy" during the annual graduation ceremony.

Mentorship teaching should be part of continuous faculty development, helping established faculty members to improve skills in mentorship. Institutions should establish protected time for discussion between faculty involved in global health work, and guidelines for management of the risks, benefits, ethics and preparation required for clinical work, both in local and distant communities. Faculty mentors should be recognized for participation in such a forum for discussion as part of their faculty development.

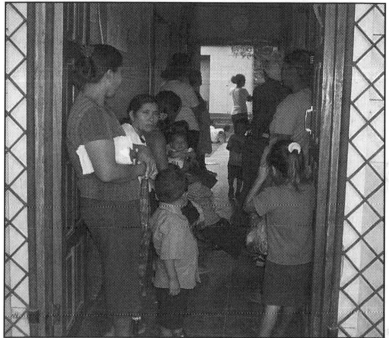

The clinic doorway in Coperna, RAAN, Nicaragua during a Tufts University School of Medicne collaborative clinic with the Nicaraguan National Health Ministry (MINSA) and international NGO Bridges to Community. (Photo credit: Jack Chase.)

Initiating and Structuring Global Health Mentorships

Strategies for initiating mentorship relationships – whether formal or informal - is rarely addressed in the literature. While formal mentor-mentee relationship programs exist in many forms, global health-specific mentorship is in its early stages. Informal mentorship in global health seems anecdotally more common. In *Sambunjak et al.*, analysis of four studies suggests that self identification of mentors was generally perceived to be beneficial, allowing a more comfortable and effective relationship to develop.

There are formal mechanisms to facilitate effective informal mentorships. Programs can create group events for residents and faculty working in global health, or formally introduce certain faculty and residents with similar interests. It would be helpful for programs to establish a list of resident and faculty interests, so that individuals and institutions might indentify potential partners.[2,6,8] Other mechanisms include rewarding faculty for being mentors, whether it be in recognition, remuneration or time built into their schedules. Some faculty may feel more empowered to mentor if they are openly appreciated for sharing their expertise and building institutional capacity.

Formal or informal mentor pairs may consider creating a shared mentorship "agreement" or contract. The content for this agreement may include frequency of meetings and mentorship timelines, modality of meetings (phone, email or in person), expectations for the mentorship and objectives, as well as frequency of revisiting the agreement.

Regarding mentorship agreements, the World Health Organization recently created MENTOR-VIP, a mentoring pilot project. MENTOR-VIP addresses the lack of resources and skills focused on the global burden of disease due to unintentional or intentional injury. The project aims to build global capacity for injury and violence prevention through mentoring. In order to help solidify mentor-mentee relationships, each pair develops and signs an individualized "mentorship accord." Preliminary evaluations from MENTOR-VIP support the critical importance of effective and regular communication between the mentor and mentee. Challenges to communication include language barriers, time zone and geographic differences, cultural differences and managing and setting clear expectations. Early evaluation also emphasized ongoing review of the relationship by mentor and mentee to ensure its utility for both parties involved.

The time commitment necessary for successful mentorship experiences is varied and highly individual. Preparation and support for a specific elective block or project may be finite, e.g. intensive meetings during a timeframe of several months. Mentorship centered around a specific project should involve preparation, problem-solving and feedback during project, and opportunities for debriefing afterward. Specific global health competencies, including knowledge-base, skill sets, and ethics, are described in other chapters in this text, In contrast to mentorship focused on a specific project, career guidance may involved less frequent meetings which are continuous over several years.

Specific Considerations for Mentorship in Global Health Rotations

Faculty mentors may play an important role in helping residents structure for clinical training experiences. The impact of effective mentorship around clinical, educational or research electives may have long lasting effects on career choice and future practice.

Mentors should be aware of the opportunities available to residents and trainees. Tremendous variation exists in the types and locations of possible training sites, which may include those directly affiliated with their institution or sites connected to other extramural health organizations. Residents and trainees may choose a site independently for specific reasons (geographical, cultural, clinical interests, etc.) Mentors should compile a database of faculty contacts and affiliations, and feedback about rotations or projects undertaken by previous residents. These contacts and feedback can be very useful to mentees considering future training sites. Faculty mentors should also be familiar with institutional requirements for resident electives regarding scheduling, educational goals, and any restrictions imposed by the program on choice of site and duration of elective.

There are numerous considerations when choosing a site. It should be emphasized that global health encompasses training and practice in both local and international communities (see Chapter 9: Global Health at Home.) Faculty mentors should engage trainees in open discussion about previous clinical experience, short-term and career goals, personal considerations, and skill-sets (linguistic, cultural, educational, clinical) in order to help guide selection of training sites. The following list of questions may be helpful for mentors and trainees regarding global health training experiences. (Specifically regarding international work, additional considerations can be found in Chapter 7: Lessons Learned – Rotation Planning Advice):

- Where do you want to go? Do you have a specific country, region or community in mind?
- Do you see yourself in an urban or a rural setting? In an inpatient or an office-based experience? Would you prefer a research experience?
- Are there specific learning objectives you want to achieve? (e.g. a resident interested in HIV care should be guided toward a site where HIV prevalence is high enough to gain significant exposure within a short period of time.)
- Do you speak another language that would be of benefit in a clinical setting? Are you seeking to improve language skills through immersion?
- What is your ethnic and cultural background, and does it influence your choice of potential training opportunities?
- Consider the safety and political stability of the site. What level of risk are you comfortable with? (By extension, what level of risk is the institution comfortable with?)
- Different communities have different degrees of resources availability – electricity, running water, access to internet/communication, etc. Which resources, if any, are critical to your educational goals? Which, if any, are important for your personal goals?

- How much time is available for planning? (Consider beginning this discussion as much as a year in advance, as some sites may fill up early or require privileging, VISA clearance, community partner identification, etc.)
- Do you have any health issues, dietary restrictions, etc. that would impact site choice?
- If the rotation is away from the home community, are you planning to bring your family, spouse or partner along?

The mentor must also take into account other important considerations from an institutional point of view. These include:

- Identification/availability of an on-site mentor. What level of supervision will the resident have? What clinical activities will be expected of the resident?
- Available funds and estimated budget
- Can clear communication with the on-site mentor be established prior to the rotation, in order to guide expectations and preparation?
- Are there residents who have rotated at the site before? What resources and needs have been identified regarding the site in consideration?

Evaluation of Mentorship

Mentorship evaluation is challenging, and seven recent peer-reviewed articles on mentorship cite the need for evaluation strategies based on tangible measurable outcomes. *Buddeberg-Fischer and Herta* conducted a Medline review of formal mentoring programs for students and physicians, and concluded that the majority of programs lack concrete structure as well as short and long-term evaluation strategies.[11] Similarly, *Gusic et al.,* conducted workshops called "The Mentorship Toolbox: How to build better mentors and mentoring programs" at three annual meetings of the Pediatric Academic Society. With over 100 participants, there was unanimous agreement that measurable outcomes must be used to demonstrate success of mentorship programs. Suggested outcomes and measurement tools include self-evaluation, focus groups, retention data and data on number of scholarly projects and promotions to measure satisfaction, growth, productivity and success within the program.

Three recent peer-reviewed articles discussed specific tools and strategies to evaluate mentorship programs based on tangible, measurable outcomes.

Berk et al. reported the findings of an *ad hoc* faculty mentoring committee established at the John Hopkins School of Nursing. This committee formed in order to set measurable mentor roles and responsibilities and develop new tools to evaluate the effectiveness of mentorship. They identified 12 measurable roles and responsibilities for the mentor:

- commits to mentoring
- provides resources, experts, and source materials in the field
- offers guidance and direction regarding professional issues
- provides timely, clear, and comprehensive feedback to mentee's questions
- encourages mentee's ideas and work
- provides constructive and useful critiques of the mentee's work
- respects mentee's uniqueness and his or her contributions
- challenges the mentee to expand his or her abilities
- appropriately acknowledges contributions of mentee
- shares success and benefits of the products and activities with mentee

Based on these 12 competency areas for the mentor, the authors developed "The Mentorship Effectiveness Scale". It consists of a series of 12 questions each utilizing a 6 point agree-disagree Likert scale. Each question corresponds to one of the 12 roles and responsibilities of the mentor. To complement this scale, the authors also developed the mentorship profile questionnaire to describe the nature of the mentoring relationship. A copy of both tools can be found in their article. The authors also call for more strategies and tools to evaluate the effectiveness of mentoring.

Rogers et al. developed a quantitative instrument to measure domains of the mentee's experience in a mentorship program.[12] They demonstrate statistical evidence in support of the tool, which was tested on 96 faculty members from one medical department. The proposed measurement tool has 27 items which follow a 5 point Likert-type scale. A full copy of the instrument can be found in the article.

The student-run Global Health Mentorship Project (GHMP) (ghmp.cfms.org or mentorship@cfms.org), having matched over 250 medical students across Canada with mentors in global health over four years, uses multiple techniques to formally and informally evaluate mentorships. Informally, each mentorship pair is assigned to a GHMP liaison, who conducts regular follow-up with the pair to ensure the mentorship is continuing smoothly. Often, this liaison, in conjunction with the rest of the GHMP team, provides learning resources for the mentorship pair to use in their discussions. Formally, each mentee completes pre- and post-mentorship surveys that address demographics, experience level in global health, expectations, level of commitment. The surveys also use Likert scales to evaluate pre- and post-mentorship knowledge of intramural and extramural global health electives, knowledge about learning and career resources in global health, and knowledge of networks and professional contacts in global health. There are additional quantitative and qualitative questions for the mentee to assess the subjective success of the mentorship and of the GHMP.

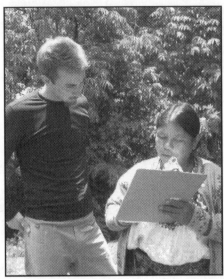

UCSF CNM student and Global Health Clinical Scholar KC Bly teaching newborn gestational age assessment techniques to Jovita, a Guatemalan traditional birth attendant. (Photo credit: Christina Ha.)

Conclusions

Mentorship in global health is an area of growing research and interest. A significant body of literature supports the importance of mentorship in medical education. Evidence is still needed to evaluate effective means of initiation, structure and monitoring for global health mentorship. Peer-reviewed literature specific to global health mentorship would be a welcome addition to current literature. In the interim, residency programs incorporating global health streams are encouraged to creatively and pragmatically include mentorship in strategies to improve global health education. Individuals committed to global health work have much to contribute by actively seeking to mentor students and residents, as well as seeking mentorship themselves. Through continuous learning, discussion and exploration we can continue to enhance our contributions to global health.

References

[1]Berk, R., Berg, J., R.Mortimer, Walton-Moss, B., & Yeo, T. (2005). Measuring the Effectiveness of Faculty Mentoring Relatoinships. *Academic Medicine*, *80* (1), 66-71.

[2] Thorndyke, L., Gusic, M., & Milner, R. (2008). Functional Mentoring: A practical approach with multilevel outcomes. *Journal of Continuing Education in the Health Professions*, 28 (3), 157-164.

[3] Koplan JP, Bond TC, Merson MH, Reddy KS, Rodriguez MH, Sewankambo NK, et al. Towards a common definition of global health. *Lancet*, 2009; 373: 1993-5.

[4] Rose GL, et al. Informal Mentoring Between Faculty and Medical Students. Academic Medicine, 2005. 80 (4): 344-8.

[5] Jackson, V., Palepu, A., Szalacha, L., & Caswell, C. (2003). Having the "right chemistry": A qualitative study of mentoring in academic medicine. *Academic Medicine*, 28 (3), 328-334.

[6] Sambunjak, D., Straus, S., & Marusic, A. (2009, November 19). A systematic review of qualatative research on the meaning and characteristics of mentoring in academic medicine. *J Gen Intern Med*. Published Online.

[7] Zerzan, J., Hess, R., Schur, E., R.Phillips, & N.Rigotti. (2009). Making the Most of Mentors: A guide for mentees. *Academic Medicine*, 84 (1), 140-4.

[8] Straus, S., Chatur, F., & Taylor, M. (2009). Issues in the Mentor–Mentee Relationship in Academic medicine- a qualatative study. *Academic medicine*, 84 (1), 135-139.

[9] Gusic, M., Zenni, E., Ludwig, S., & First, L. (2010). Strategies to Design an Effective Mentorship Program. *Journal of Pediatrics*, 156 (2).

[10] Rammani, S., Gruppen, L., & Kachur, E. (2006). Twelve Tips for Developing Effective Mentors. *Medical Teacher*, 28 (5), 404-8.

[11] Buddeberg-Fischer, B., & Herta, K. (2006). Formal Mentorship Programs for Medical students and doctors: a Review of the mediline literature. *Medical Teacher*, 28 (3), 248-56.

[12] Rogers, J., & F. Marconi Monteiro, A. N. (2008). Toward Measuringt he Domains of Mentoring. *Family Medicine*, 40 (4), 259-53.

-- American Medical Student Association Toolkit for Going Abroad. Accessed online on July 30, 2009 at : http://www.amsa.org/global/ih/toolkit.cfm

-- Clarke, K. Toolkit for Medical Visits Abroad. 2006. Available on line from the American Academy of Pediatrics Section on International Child Health at: http://www.aap.org/Sections/ich/resources.htm

-- Davis, C et al. Planning and Preparation, in The GHEC Guidebook: Advising Medical Students and Residents for International Health Experiences. Global Health Education Consortium, 2000.

-- Dueger, C and O'Callahan, C. Working in International Child Health, second edition. American Academy of Pediatrics, 2008.

-- Waugh, JL. Faculty Mentoring Guide – VCU School of Medicine. Virginia Commonwealth University, 2002. Accessed July 30, 2009 at: http://www.medschool.vcu.edu/facultyaffairs/career_dev/facultymentoringguide/fm guide.pdf

-- A.Hyder, D.Meddings, & A.Bachani. (2009). MENTOR-VIP: Piloting a Global Mentoring Program for Injury and Violence Prevention. *Academic Medicine*, *84* (6), 793-96.

-- Koskinen, L., & Tossavainen, K. (2003). Charactersistics of intercultural mentoring- a mentor perspective. *Nurse Education Today , 23*, 278-285.

*Tom Bodenheimer, Jack Chase, Kevin Grumbach, L. Masae Kawamura,
James H. McKerrow, Stephanie Taché, Anthony Valdini*

Introduction

Historically, global health programs in highly resourced nations have
focused on underserved communities in international, often rural, settings
(see Chapter 1: Introduction to Global Health.) More recently, allied health
educators and medical professionals have begun to explore challenges
common to both local and global health – poverty, infrastructure deficits,
low health literacy, addiction, traumatic injury, cultural and linguistic
barriers, and increasing prevalence of chronic diseases such as hypertension
and diabetes. The disciplines which compose the foundation of global
health – medicine, sociology, psychology, community organizing,
engineering, research and bench science, humanities, and others – are
powerful tools to address these challenges in any community.

Graduate medical training programs often serve marginalized local
communities faced with challenges that reflect global trends. These local
communities are meaningful potential partners for bidirectional exchange.
Relationships between GME programs and community partners strive to
improve community wellness and local capacity while providing service
and learning opportunities for medical professionals. Practice and
refinement of skills in home communities may improve readiness for
addressing barriers to health in international settings; and conversely, work
in distant communities can teach valuable lessons for use in home
environments.

The following passages are written by a group of physicians,
research scientists, educators and community organizers who work
primarily in the United States with diseases, social issues and infrastructural
inadequacies of global importance. Each of the authors was asked "How
does your work locally reflect a global health issue?" and "What skills can
training health professionals learn through work in local communities which
can be applied in international settings?" Their responses highlight
universal themes, and describe strategies applicable to global health training
and practice.

Geography, Borders, Reservations and Isolation
Anthony Valdini, MD, MS

*Dr. Valdini is a senior faculty member at the Lawrence Family Medicine
Residency (see chapter 10 for a program profile.) Over the course of his
career he has worked in many under-resourced communities, both in the*

United States and abroad, including as the medical director of the Navajo
Nation Health Foundation, the co-director of a public health collaboration
with the Nicaraguan MINSA in rural Northeastern Nicaragua, and as a
family physician and medical educator in the diverse and underserved
community of Lawrence, Massachusetts.

Of course, people from developing countries do sometimes bring diseases with them as they travel from their natal community to the United States. We have seen dengue, malaria, leprosy, tuberculosis and typhoid fever in persons recently "off the plane." These exotic diseases are usually devastating and acute. They are impossible to ignore and are best handled in the hospital. But the simple fact of being in a new community alone and without support is a more sinister and chronic risk factor for physical and psychological illness, and its effects aren't always realized.

One of the most important lessons we, as providers and fellow community members, have learned by working with diasporic communities is that loneliness is a risk factor for having a myocardial infarction and dying from it, as well as suffering a simple URI, and social capital is in short supply in many immigrant communities.[1,2,3] People leave their families and support systems behind in search of a better life. Sometimes, even though economic circumstances improve, (e.g., monthly welfare benefits in Lawrence, Massachusetts for a family of 4 are greater than the average yearly income in the Dominican Republic,) social isolation leads to loneliness and sometimes depression. This isolation is reflected in patterns of medical system utilization in persons who are lonely. We have found that in our practice, consisting of a majority of immigrants from the Dominican Republic and Puerto Rico, lonely people visit the emergency room, the labor deck for false labor and the clinic more often than their counterparts even when controlling for level of illness.

Social capital is related to trust of an individual and consists of generosity by others based this trust.[4] The trust is often extended to a person's neighbors and family, thus binding communities together. When a person leaves their home community in the hope of improved quality of life, they trade a portion, sometimes all, of their social capital for the potential of a "new life". The situation where a person knew and trusted their neighbors and could ask them for help, changes to a new situation far from home, where they have no personal connection and are on their own. New immigrants struggle with questions like "Can I borrow cab fare to bring my daughter to the ER? Who can watch my other children while I do so?" "Does anyone I know own tools I can borrow to fix my plumbing?" "How about a co-pay for antibiotics?"

In addition to a lack of social capital, there are multiple items that can contribute to immigrants' alienation and the challenge of transition. In the case of immigration to the United States, a short list of these challenges includes the lack of English language skills, low levels of literacy and numeracy, inadequate money and insurance, temporary or absent documentation for legal status and difficulty finding employment. Surprisingly, despite an improved standard of living whether through wages or public assistance, "relative poverty" can lead to alienation and, similar to unemployment, a lack of self worth.

A critical element of caring for vulnerable populations is a sensitivity to the effect of poverty on health. The trickiest part of cultural competence isn't the differences between language or customs, it is the problem of the dealing with attitudes and expectations that are bred from poverty. Most physicians are not familiar with the behaviors engendered by being raised in abject poverty. Values are often different toward things like education, for example: roughly one-third of the Lawrence High School student population turns over each year with migration back and forth to the islands. It is difficult for many of our patients to understand that they can actually earn a 6 figure income through education and training in the US.

Social norms differ in communities with differing levels of resources. Appointments are usually unheard of in many less resourced communities, therefore they mean little; alternatively, one's place in line means everything. Additionally, in their previous home communities many of our patients came to understand that offices have neither diagnostic equipment nor medications to treat them. Folk beliefs and remedies exist and are viable sometimes preferable alternatives and are utilized prior to seeking out "western medicine". These treatments may include teas, herbs, ceremonies, charms, and even Vicks Vapo-Rub.

Prior to immigration, in resource limited settings, many of our patients were forced to choose between economic ruination and medical treatment, sometimes with life in the balance. Many recent immigrants are not accustomed to subsidized full-spectrum care, where a person, if acutely ill "enough," can receive care without regard to payment (by law). Because our immigrant patients have seen loved ones die due to lack of care they will often go to ER in lieu of the office wishing to get the biggest and best care for their families.

While many people, both health care professionals and others, think of global health and limited resources as related more to rural communities, urban poverty is just as damaging to health outcomes. With issues of stark intraurban economic differences, inadequate space to live and play in poor neighborhoods, scarcity of options for healthy nutrition, gangs and violence, drug and alcohol abuse – being poor in the city is different than in the country.

In my experience, some aspects of life and practice in an urban, underserved community are opposite from life on a reservation. On the reservation, *the physician* is in a diaspora, far away physically and socially from his family, culture, and most critically, "class," meaning educational level. In a visual example, at my first department head meeting at Sage Memorial hospital, I was the only adult male in the room NOT wearing a baseball cap (indoors). Try to picture that in your local hospital's grand rounds.

Successful long-term learners to come to a peace with being outsiders, they realize that they are from "away" and don't try to "go native" e.g. wearing buckskins and a large knife on your belt. They will make friends with locals, but acknowledge that it really isn't their culture that they are witnessing and dealing with daily. My experience in the Navajo nation was shaped by strong cultural values for the Navajos I worked with, but to be sure- *they were home*. It was we who were the outsiders.

Global health is reflected in foodways, religion, family dynamics, cultural history and aspirations of the people we serve. Rarely, as they travel from their natal home to a new community, our patients bring a disease along with them – dengue, scrofula, TB – but more commonly they become "infected" with chronic illnesses from exposure to our habits: smoking, drinking, obesity. We may be knowledgeable about our local geography, demographics and health issues, but unfamiliar with the unique and diverse characteristics of the communities and populations we treat. If one wishes to work with different cultures and can do so, learning the language spoken by community members can open many doors into the thoughts and expectations of your patients. In addition to language, leaving the clinic or hospital, getting to know people and asking them (gently) about their lives and aspirations and families really is a valuable education. These two pieces of cultural competency are invaluable in learning about any community, in your home town, or across the globe.

"Neglected Tropical Diseases" are not always tropical, and should not be neglected
James McKerrow, MD, PhD

Dr. McKerrow is the director of the Sandler Center for Basic Research in Parasitic Diseases at the University of California San Francisco, where he leads a consortium of research laboratories searching for new and effective treatments for infectious diseases largely neglected by resourced nations and by the global pharmaceutical industry.

Neglected tropical diseases (NTDs) are a designation given to a group of parasitic diseases by the U.S. National Institutes of Health and the World Health Organization. Neglected tropical diseases include schistosomiasis, leishmaniasis, African sleeping sickness, Chagas' disease, and malaria. They are called "neglected" because although they affect hundreds of millions of people worldwide, they are largely "neglected" by the pharmaceutical industry. This is because they are primarily diseases of poor people in poor regions of the world. As such, developing drugs or vaccines against these diseases do not represent a viable market for the industry.

If you choose to work in countries in which these diseases are endemic, you will see that they are major health problems throughout the tropical world. However, with economic globalization and immigration, these diseases have also become "local." For example, Chagas' disease is the leading cause of heart disease in Latin America, and is caused by a single cell protozoan parasite, *Trypanosoma cruzi*. It is estimated that somewhere between eight to 12 million people are infected with the parasite, with over 80 million at risk. Recently, this disease has been identified in the United States with increasing frequency. First, it was found in a significant percentage of blood received for blood transfusions in U.S. blood centers. As a result, all blood must now be tested for the parasite. Secondly, the disease is clearly a problem in the U.S. immigrant population from Latin America. This is obviously both a health problem and a political problem in that anti-immigration literature can brand immigrants as "bringing" Chagas' disease to this country. As a result, the extent of Chagas' disease in the United States is largely hidden because people are afraid to access healthcare facilities for fear of being deported. It would behoove modern-day anti-immigration proponents to realize that historically the same criticism was made over the past century of immigrants from Europe for "bringing in" tuberculosis to the United States.

Chagas' disease is also an endemic problem in domestic dogs in the United States, particularly in the southwest, where transmission from the insect vector occurs in exactly the same way it is transmitted to humans in Latin America. This raises the possibility that local transmission from the insect vector could occur in the United States as well.

Another example of a "tropical disease" that can be local is malaria. Even if you choose to practice medicine in the United States, you will undoubtedly see cases of malaria in individuals who have been tourists in tropical regions of the world, or military personnel stationed overseas. What is more important to recognize is that malaria was in fact an endemic problem in the United States at least into the 1930s. "Old timers" from Charleston, South Carolina will tell you that wealthy families would leave Charleston during the "malaria season," and spend their summers in the mountains of North Carolina. The malaria zone was not only the warm and humid southeast, but virtually all major waterways, including the large rivers that traverse the Midwest. Malaria was a significant problem for Lewis and Clark during their expedition, and even was a problem in states like Indiana that are not considered "tropical." Control of malaria in the United States was almost exclusively due to the use of insecticides like DDT. The point is that if the mosquito vectors of malaria are not kept under control, malaria could certainly re-emerge in the United States at any time. All physicians practicing in the U.S. should be vigilant for the re-emergence of this and other parasitic diseases.

By developing a knowledge base and a clinical eye for these diseases, health care providers not only improve their care of local patients, but build a new skill set for international settings. The burden of "tropical" disease among local populations, even in highly resourced settings, is a constant reminder of the interconnectedness of global health concerns in local and distant communities.

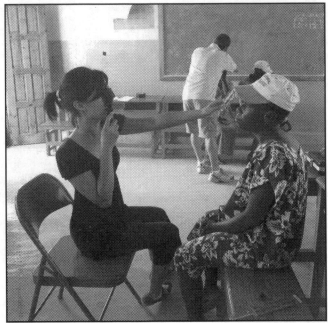

Peony Tam, Western University of Health Sciences College of Optometry second year student, performing retinoscopy in Silegue, Haiti. (Photo credit: Kierstyn Napier-Dovorany.)

Teamlets and Health Coaches – Improving Primary Care through Community Health Liaisons
Tom Bodenheimer, MD

Dr. Bodenheimer is a professor of Family and Community Medicine at the University of California San Francisco, and the co-director of the UCSF Center for Excellence in Primary Care. Dr. Bodenheimer's research focuses on primary care improvement and innovation, especially related to chronic diseases such as diabetes and hypertension, and is informed by his over three decades as a clinician in solo practice.

Primary care is often viewed as a team-based activity. Yet many practices have experienced difficulty implementing high-performing teams. The larger the team, the more time and energy are spent communicating among team members and the greater the probability of fumbled handoffs. Smaller teams may have advantages, especially in resource-limited settings.

Years ago, primary care practices consisted solely of a doctor and a nurse, often working together for many years. They trusted each other, they worked out a division of labor, and the patients trusted them both. This was the original *teamlet*. This traditional model survives today in small primary care offices, though in many cases the nurse has been replaced by a medical assistant, who may be trained as a health coach.

The primary function of a health coach is to assist patients to gain the knowledge, skills, and confidence to self-manage their chronic conditions. Specifically, health coaches:

- help patients set agendas for the clinician visit
- make sure patients understand what their clinician wants them to do
- determine whether patients agree with their care plans
- provide support to patients' efforts in adopting healthy behaviors
- assist patients to improve medication understanding and adherence
- function as a cultural bridge, point of access, and support for their patients

Health coaches have correlates in international settings and are known by many titles including *promotora*, and *accompagnateur*. Healthcare teams may also include other types of clinicians, including physician assistants (see Chapter 11: Physician Assistants in Global Health.)

San Francisco General Hospital's Family Health Center (FHC), a residency teaching clinic, has explored the use of small, two-person teamlets. A teamlet consists of a clinician (physician, nurse practitioner or physician assistant) and health coach. Ideally, the two people work together every day, sharing responsibility for the health of their patient panel.

In the ideal setting, each clinic session would begin with a teamlet huddle to discuss the day's patients. By going over the scheduled patients, the teamlet can anticipate how to best address patient concerns, and share the burden of non-clinical patient issues. For example, the teamlet decides which patients the health coach should help by setting the visit agenda, or assisting with medication review prior to the visit. During a visit, the health coach can take notes, make copies of documents, and ensure that the visit runs smoothly. After the visit, the health coach "closes the loop," making sure patients understand what the physician said, explaining medication purpose and dosing, and developing behavior-change action plans with patients to manage chronic conditions. Phone or home visit follow-up between clinic visits is essential to inquire about subjective changes in the patient's symptoms, to check up on behavior-change action plans and to determine whether the patient is taking medications as prescribed.

The health coach is the bridge between the patient and clinician. Health coaching is especially important for vulnerable populations with poor access to services and cultural and language barriers. Health coaches trained from the community can offer ethnically and language concordant care for their patients, establishing added investment between patients and their care teams. They can improve the experience and efficacy of the solo clinician as well as in a group practice environment. In resource limited settings, health coaches can serve both in the clinic and also as physician extenders to geographically isolated communities. The training of health coaches also provides these individuals with a highly valuable skill set to enable employment. Many resource limited communities share similar characteristics: high rates of unemployment, high patient to provider ratios, geographic distance from health care, limited health literacy, and linguistic and cultural barriers between community members and treating physicians. Health coaches can be a valuable resource to improve wellness in communities facing any or all of these challenges, both at home and abroad.

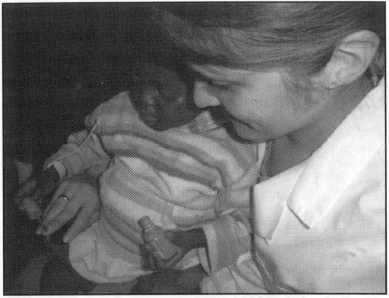

Megan Little, first year medical student at Wright State University Boonshoft School of Medicine, bonds with seven-year-old Sanelisiwe over nail polish at Raleigh Fitkin Memorial Hospital in Manzini, Swaziland.
(Photograph by Alicia Boyd)

Tuberculosis: A Window into Global Public Health

Dr. Masae Kawamura is the Tuberculosis Controller and Medical Director for the Tuberculosis Section of the San Francisco Department of Public Health. She is the co-principle investigator of the Francis J. Curry National Tuberculosis Center at the University of California San Francisco, and an active investigator in the Centers for Disease Control Tuberculosis

148

Trials Consortium. In addition to her work in the United States, she has worked in Bhutan as the Physician-in-Chief of the Tuberculosis and Infectious Disease Ward and consultant to the country's National Tuberculosis Programme.

As the result of the worldwide impact and endemicity of tuberculosis (TB,) TB control in the United States provides a window to the world of global public health. One third of the human population is infected with TB. Outside highly resourced nations, tuberculosis is one of the largest single causes of morbidity and mortality in the world, accounting for nearly 9 million new infections and 2 million deaths yearly.[5] TB is a major factor in nations challenged by poverty, especially those with high rates of HIV, and it affects people at all levels of society. It influences national, continental, and global policy and healthcare decision making. Within the borders of more highly resourced nations, such as the United States, TB provides a perspective on the interaction between resource scarcity and illness, as a disease of poverty and of migration.

High rates of TB infection among new immigrants and special local populations reflect lower standards of living and limited health care resources. Patterns of migration and international TB transmission are observed in growing multi-drug resistance rates found among newcomers in California. Changing patterns of immigration and new diasporic populations that we see in our TB Clinic give insight into the impact of current global trends, such as famine, economic deprivation, and the impact of war. Co-infection of TB and HIV among domestically born patients presents the challenge of populations with high levels of endemic disease in local communities; and the higher rate of TB among the homeless reminds us of the connection between poverty, deprivation and illness, which is present even in highly resourced nations.

In providing medical care for immigrants with tuberculosis, one immediately recognizes the disparities in health delivery, safety regulations and standards of care between our country and those abroad. Rates and patterns of drug resistance in new immigrants are due in part to lax policies in home countries regarding the purchase of antibiotics, including TB drugs, without a prescription or physician oversight. Additionally, many countries with endemic TB have inadequate healthcare workforce to ensure complete treatment for infected patients. Patients presenting to the United States with newly diagnosed culture-positive TB may have been missed prior to migration by 3 negative smears in their home country, because the standard WHO strategy does not include cultures.

The local epidemiology of immigrants is a snapshot of epidemiology in their countries of origin. As an example, the recent increasing trend of simultaneous diagnosis of HIV and TB in Mexican women new to the United States is a tip-off to converging epidemics and unchecked HIV transmission in Mexico. TB patients also represent the interaction between disease and global economic trends. As commercialization and industry spread to even isolated global communities, the impact of tobacco marketing in developing countries increases the already high incidence of smoking. This is a complicating factor in TB outcomes as smoking is now a recognized risk factor for TB infection and disease.

Domestically, poverty, substance abuse and mental illness are risk factors for poor TB outcomes, and rates of TB are disproportionately high among racial and ethnic minorities. Disenfranchisement from the health system likely plays a role in this relationship, and presents a continuing target for domestic public health efforts.

Practicing public health in the US gives an appreciation for our domestic health care infrastructure, standards of care, guidelines for infection control, and fair public health laws. We have the resources to provide the highest quality of care for communicable diseases, such as tuberculosis, to any and all affected people. This care usually comes at no cost to the patient, and care for public health problems like TB is not rationed. Adequate resources and mature, patient-centered care enable TB patients to adhere to their treatment. We are able to provide transportation to the clinic, temporary lodging for the homeless during treatment, food to the poor that cannot work because they are contagious, and thereby foster relationships that build trust and confidence in the disenfranchised.

Universally, treating a TB patient until completion is directly related to relationship building through mutual respect and trust. As in the care of people from all communities, knowledge of health attitudes and cultural literacy are critical to provider success. Kindness, reliability and a respectful attitude are key staff attributes, essential in working with foreign-born populations and local communities. As we care for the next generations of people affected by tuberculosis, efforts toward global TB control and more equitable resource allocation may allow for future gains in outcomes for people from all nations.

A New Paradigm for Global Health Training: Reconciling Domestic Health Disparities with International Health
Kevin Grumbach MD and Stephanie Taché MD, MPH

Dr. Grumbach is Professor and Chair of the UCSF Department of Family and Community Medicine. His research focuses on primary care physician supply in underserved communities, racial and ethnic diversity in the health professions and domestic health disparities. Dr. Taché is an assistant clinical professor at the University of California San Francisco in the Department of Family and Community Medicine at San Francisco General Hospital. She is co-director for the UCSF Masters in Global Health Sciences course on Chronic Diseases. Among other topics, her research has focused on workforce shortage and capacity building in under-resourced nations, and medical education in global health. The following passage is from an upcoming article by the authors.

Interest in global health has surged in recent years among medical students and physicians in residency training in the US. At our own institution (UCSF), over 50% of entering medical students express an interest in global health. Students and residents view international electives in developing nations as particularly enriching experiences. This growing student interest in global health presents challenges for finding ways to provide meaningful experiences for students abroad without creating additional burdens on severely under-resourced host institutions. The traditional episodic format of a four to six week clinical rotation at a clinic or hospital in a developing nation runs the risk of becoming a form of "medical tourism," taxing local training resources without offering prospects of long-term returns to the host country. One approach to mitigating the phenomenon of medical tourism is for home institutions to develop coordinated and ongoing partnerships with international sites, with attention to long-term funding and sustainable relationships between partner institutions.[6]

Of equal importance is requiring that trainees process their international experiences in a manner that allows them to translate lessons learned abroad to local U.S. settings, emphasizing commonalities in the health problems facing domestic and international communities and in the approaches needed to successfully address health disparities. Many students interested in global health also have an interest in caring for domestic underserved populations.[7,8,9] Connecting curricula in domestic health disparities to experiences in global health has been a missing link in most global health training programs. There is important overlap in the approaches and skills needed to address the health problems of underserved populations internationally and domestically. Cross cutting skills include health policy analysis, cultural competency, leadership skills, how to engage with communities, and understanding the role of socioeconomic status in disease and health. Highlighting domestic health issues with global ramifications helps demonstrate the extent to which health and disease are intertwined around the world. We describe three health issues with complex political, economic and social dynamics present in both the developing world and the United States. These examples are intended to illustrate the ways in which curricula in global health could emphasize the connectivity between global and local health issues.

Malnutrition: Undernourished and Overfed

Malnutrition most often refers to undernutrition resulting from the lack of sufficient nutrients to maintain optimal health. There are an estimated 800 million people suffering from undernutrition worldwide and it is typically associated with extreme poverty in developing countries. Undernutrition is estimated to contribute to more than one third of the disease burden in developing countries.[10] However, malnutrition also encompasses the phenomenon of over nutrition resulting from excessive intake of specific nutrients. Some have estimated that there are now more overweight people across the world than undernourished people.[11] The number of overweight people has topped one billion, of which 300 million are obese. The United States has one of the highest rates of obesity in the world, with rates increasing sharply over the past 30 years. Obese individuals are at heightened risk to develop type II diabetes, hypertension, osteoarthritis, dyslipidemia and coronary heart disease. Attention to the upstream factors leading to obesity in the US requires focusing on the social factors promoting poor nutrition and inadequate physical activity such as tax subsidies for agri-business, fast food culture, urban planning, and transportation systems.

Both under- and over nutrition have links to the problem of food security – the availability of safe, nutritious, and socially acceptable food. Food insecurity may be chronic, seasonal, or temporary, and it may occur at the household, regional, or national level. In developing countries, the root causes of food insecurity include poverty, war and civil conflict, natural disasters, corruption, barriers to trade, low levels of education, and national policies that do not promote equal access to food for all. In the United States, the primary causes of food insecurity are poverty and public subsidies for mass-produced, agricultural mono-crops such as corn, which render high caloric, processed foods less expensive than more nutrient dense, perishable food such as fruits and vegetables. The US has also promoted these same agricultural policies in its food exports and approach to international aid, to the detriment of agricultural diversity, sustainable farming, and indigenous food security in developing nations. As Western dietary styles and food habits continue to be adopted around the world, the obesity epidemic remains one of the major unresolved global health issues disproportionately affecting the United States, but now also rising in prevalence in developing nations. To understand the contextual factors which lead to different forms of malnutrition, medical students must be versed in the food policies that influence the type of food available to affected populations globally.

Youth Violence and Injury

Violence and injury is another complex global health problem. Causing over 5 million deaths every year, violence and injuries account for 9% of global mortality -- as many deaths as from HIV, malaria and tuberculosis combined. There have been more than 160 wars and armed conflicts since 1945, almost all in developing countries. The nature of armed conflict has changed substantially over time and more than 90% of these are internal rather than between sovereign states.[12] Violence across the world takes a disproportionate toll on the health of young people. Eight of the 15 leading causes of death for people ages 15 to 29 years are injury-related and three of these are intentional injuries from homicide, suicide, and poisoning. Youth injury caused by firearms in developing countries has increased with greater availability of weapons over the past decades. A study of former child soldiers in Africa found that over 90% had witnessed a shooting, more than half had killed someone, and one-third suffered from post-traumatic stress disorder (PTSD).

This pattern of gun-related violence and injury has its parallels in the U.S. Juvenile firearm violence became common in many U.S. cities during the 1990s with the rise of gangs and remains a persistent and vexing problem. Among 10 to 24 year olds, homicide is the leading cause of death for African Americans, the second leading cause of death for Hispanics, and the third leading cause of death for American Indians, Alaska Natives, and Asian/Pacific Islanders. Although the reach of violence in the US does not match the horrific scale of armed conflicts in parts of the world, some inner city communities in the US have endemic levels of violence that create the same type of pervasively traumatic social environments found in communities ravaged by war. In some cities in the US, almost half of inner city youth have seen someone shot or stabbed.[13] Post Traumatic Stress Disorder (PTSD) is widely prevalent in inner city communities among victims, perpetrators, and witnesses of violence and plays a role in perpetuating further violence.[8]

Whether the focus is on child soldiers in Africa or children drafted into gangs in US cities, violence has similar long-term health impacts and psychosocial consequences in distressed communities across the globe. Global efforts to prevent violence require an understanding of the relationships among important social determinants of violence. These efforts require multi-disciplinary approaches, involving school officials, law enforcement, social services, community organizations and local health departments. Health care professionals in all settings also must appreciate the range of health outcomes of political violence and civil conflict, particularly mental health outcomes, and gain skills in how to intervene to interrupt the cycle of violence. Curricula in global health should highlight these common themes and encourage students to apply lessons learned in international experiences to addressing issues of violence in their local neighborhoods.

Equitable Access to Health Care

A concern for equity in access to healthcare services is one of the core ethical principles of global health. To a large degree, the interest in global health among students in the US is an expression of their desire to ameliorate suffering and improve health in places where the gap between the health care "haves" and "have nots" of the world is most glaring. The US Government has also, in many instances, responded to these global inequities with compassion and generosity. An example is the role played by the Federal Government in providing resources for HIV/AIDS care and treatment in developing nations. More people in Sub-Saharan Africa have had access to highly effective anti-retrovirals at minimal charge through the Presidential Emergency Plan for AIDS Relief than from any other program.

One question that students travelling abroad for international health experiences are invariably asked by residents of other nations is why the US tolerates such extreme inequities in health care for its own citizens. In 2006, 47 million Americans were uninsured – 15.8% of the population. Lack of insurance compromises health because less preventive care is received, late presentation to care leads to more advanced disease stages and, once diagnosed, the uninsured tend to receive less therapeutic care and have higher mortality rates than insured individuals.[14] This pattern of late presentation to care and unmet medical need is seen in most developing countries where large segments of the population have limited access to healthcare, and only a small elite can afford a higher standard of care. Yet these inequities in access to care within developing nations occur in settings of impoverished national economies and highly constrained resources overall for health care. Such cannot be said of the situation in the US. US healthcare expenditures in 2005 accounted for almost 45% of the $4.4 trillion spent globally on health.[15,16]

Discussing the ethical implications of this paradox is essential for any global health apprenticeship. Curricula in global health should address issues of distributive justice in health care, and ask students to reflect not only on inequities in health and health care *between* nations, but inequities *within* nations, including our own. During experiences abroad, students should be encouraged to explore how nations with health care budgets that are a fraction of that of the US often achieve much better value for their spending and more equitable distribution of their health care resources.

A New Paradigm

Students bring diverse interests, experiences, and aspirations to their exposure to global health during their training. A distinct minority of these students will ultimately go on to long term careers stationed abroad or with a primary focus on global health. For many students, a one month elective spent in a health center in a developing nation will be their first and last hands-on experience in international health. If educational programs in global health are to avoid being exercises in medical tourism, it is imperative that these programs emphasize the links between these global experiences and issues closer to home. By exploring the commonalities of global health problems domestically and abroad, we include ourselves in the broader framework of global health, rather than casting ourselves as outsiders seeking to help others in far off places of the world with "their problems."

The complex global health issues of obesity, violence and health equity illustrate the types of problems that curricula could highlight to explore these commonalities. These topics are offered as examples, and there are many other topics that would be worthy of highlighting in global health curricula to stimulate discussion and reflection on connections between global health issues both internationally and domestically to identify cross-cutting skills in community health applicable across settings.

We believe that the approach we are recommending would have manifold benefits to global health education programs and students. If taught prior to an international placement, this type of curriculum would provide students a template to better recognize underlying health system dynamics in their host nation that resonate with familiar domestic themes. Appreciating that the US is susceptible to many of the same underlying health problems might also encourage students to approach their placements with more cultural humility. A global health education program of this type would also facilitate students' application of the lessons learned abroad to their engagement in efforts to address health disparities at home. Fundamentally, the goal of such a program would be to educate health professionals to be more effective agents to improve the health of communities and eliminate health disparities using the "think globally, act locally" approach—no matter where on the globe they might be.

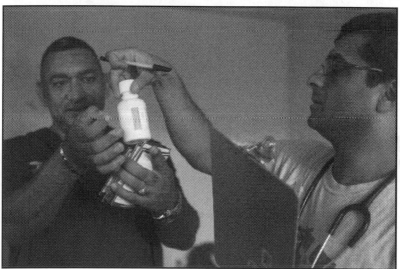

Family Physician Dr. Ayaz Madraswalla discusses dosages with Dr. Jose Yuñen, from Puerto Plata, Dominican Republic, at Health Horizons International's clinic in nearby Severet. (Photo credit: Rachel Geylin.)

References

[1] Orth-Gomer K, Unden A, Edwards M. Social isolation and mortality in ischemic heart disease. *Acta Med Scand* 1988;224:205-15.

[2] Berkman L, Leo-summers L, Horowiitz R. Emotional support and survival after myocardial infarction. *Ann Int Med* 1992; 117:1003-9.

[3] Cohen S, Doyle W, Skoner D, Rubin B, Gwaltney J. Social ties and susceptibility to the common cold. *JAMA* 1997;277:1940-4.

[4] Baum F. Social capital: is it good for your health? Issues for a public health agenda. *J Epidemiol Community Health* 1999;53:195-6.

[5] From the Centers for Disease Control (CDC) Tuberculosis Factsheet, available at http://www.cdc.gov/tb. Accessed December 1, 2010.

[6] Taché S, Kaaya, E., Omer, S. et al. University partnership to address the shortage of healthcare professionals in Africa. *Global Public Health.* 2008;3(2):137-148.

[7] Godkin M, Savageau J. The effect of medical students' international experiences on attitudes toward serving underserved multicultural populations. *Fam Med.* 2003 35(4):273-278.

[8] Haq C, Rothenberg D, Gjerde C, et al. New world views: preparing physicians in training for global health work. *Fam Med.* 2000 32(8):566-572.

[9] Ramsey A, Haq C, Gjerde C, et al. Career influence of an international health experience during medical school. *Fam Med.* 2004;36(6):412-416.

[10] Murray C, Lopez, A., editors. *The Global Burden of Disease, Vol. I: a comprehensive assessment of mortality and disability from diseases, injuries, and risk factors in 1990 and projected to 2020.* ; 1996.

[11] Popkin B, Gordon-Larsen D. The nutrition transition: worldwide obesity dynamics and their determinants. *International Journal of Obesity.* 2004;28:S2-S9.

[12] Summerfield D. The social, cultural and political dimensions of contemporary war. *Med Confl Surviv.* . 1997;13(1):3-25.

[13] Schwab-Stone, Kasprow W, Voyce C, et al. No safe haven: A study of violence exposure in an urban community. *Journal of the American Academy of Child and Adolescent Psychiatry.* 1995;34:1343-1352.

[14] Institute of Medicine. *Care Without Coverage - Too Little, Too Late.*: The National Academies Press; 2002.

[15] World Health Organization. *Spending on Health: A Global Overview.* Geneva 2007.

[16] National Health Expenditure summary including share of GDP, CY 1960-2006. Office of the Actuary: Data from the National Health Statistics Group.; 2007. Updated Last Updated Date. Accessed July 10, 2008.

Jack Chase, Laura Janneck, Christopher Prater and Michael Slatnick

The importance of a global focus in medical education has driven curriculum innovation in residency and fellowship training. The goal of this chapter is to present strategies for increasing global focus in graduate medical education and to highlight creativity. The chapter does not offer a comprehensive list of all training programs with global health opportunities. As discussed in Chapter 9, many of the programs mentioned in this chapter work with diverse and underserved populations in their own communities, in addition to providing opportunities for international work. This chapter is underscored by the need for each residency program to look at its unique strengths and resources to provide global health exposure. By drawing on community partners, institutional champions, and existing strengths, programs can carve out their own approach to global health which is sustainable and relevant for communities both local and abroad.

The descriptions provided in this chapter are largely in the programs' own words, and are up to date at the time of publication. Training programs continue to develop and enhance their curricula, and details can change year to year. We recommend contacting programs for the most up to date information. Additional resources for information about global health-focused programs are available at the end of the chapter.

Residency Programs

Aboriginal Family Medicine Residency

Hospital: Royal Jubilee, Victoria General Hospital
Affiliation: University of British Columbia School of Medicine
Location: Victoria, British Columbia, Canada
Year Established: 2002
Disciplines: Family Medicine
Enrollment: 4 residents per year
Website: http://www.familymed.ubc.ca/carms/sites/aboriginal.htm

Brief Overview and History
The Aboriginal Residency Program at the University of British Columbia trains physicians (both Indigenous and non-Indigenous) to become family practitioners with a subspecialty in Aboriginal Health. The program was founded in order to address inequities in the health of Aboriginal people which were highlighted in 2001 in the British Columbia Health Officer's Report, "The Health and Wellbeing of Aboriginal People in British Columbia." These inequities include the inadequate number of physicians

working with Aboriginal peoples, inadequate understanding and skills to meet the needs of Aboriginal communities, as well as inadequate number of Aboriginal doctors in the country. The program focuses on Indigenous approaches to health care, emphasizing cultural sensitivity and community involvement.

Program Goals and Objectives

The health status of Aboriginal people in Canada is poor across a spectrum of indicators and, at the same time, the Aboriginal population is growing faster than the general population. This program's aim is to train physicians with knowledge of Aboriginal health issues, foster the development of cultural competencies to work effectively with Aboriginal patients and communities, and develop a growing number of human resources who can guide others to improve the overall health of our Native people.

Curriculum Highlights and Notable Rotations

The curriculum explores topics that affect Aboriginal health, including racism, colonialism, marginalization, residential schools, and social determinants of health.

- Residents receive teachings specific to Aboriginal health one day a month including didactic formal lectures and community engagement.
- The educational program focuses on Aboriginal patients in Family Medicine and elective rotations: one month family medicine rotation in Alert Bay during the R1 year, and work in areas where Aboriginals are disproportionately represented (addictions, prison medicine, inner city) and other disciplines (emergency medicine and obstetrics)
- Residents have opportunities for interaction with elders, Aboriginal physicians and community visits are incorporated into academic sessions
- Residents receive support for attendance at Aboriginal conferences and workshops
- Teaching emphasizes understanding health in the context of the medicine wheel as well as other Aboriginal paradigms for health
- Training incorporates traditional healing practices and beliefs as well as an understanding of the importance of these practices to many First Nations
- Family medicine and first year Royal College residents are the only full time postgraduate trainees
- Residents have opportunities to partner with Canadian Aboriginal Leaders in Medicine (CALM) and Indigenous Physicians Association of Canada (IPAC.)

The program includes the following clinical rotations, which it highlights on its website.

- *Rural Rotation:* During the second year, residents must complete a minimum two-month core rotation in a rural family practice in a primarily Aboriginal community such as Bella Bella, Queen Charlotte City, Massett, Alert Bay, Inuvik, 100 Mile House, Vanderhoof, or the Central Interior Native Health Centre in Prince George. Family practice experience is balanced to provide residents with an opportunity to work with a strong and successful Aboriginal community as well as communities that are facing numerous health and social challenges.
- *Inner-City Medicine:* Second year residents complete a minimum one-month rotation in inner-city medicine at a Native Health Clinic, which will provide a link with the local public health programs.
- *Community Health:* Second year residents must complete a minimum one-month rotation in mental health community programs with an emphasis on acquiring counseling skills. This rotation can be carried out longitudinally.
- *Addiction Medicine and Prison Medicine:* In the second year, residents may elect to complete a one-month rotation in addictions or prison medicine. Aboriginal people are over-represented in the Canadian prison system. Prison inmates often have concurrent illnesses as well as unmet health needs, occurring in a group with increased high-risk behaviors. This rotation will provide an introduction to these specialized health care programs and provide an opportunity for residents to address some of the unmet needs.

Faculty
Residents are taught by physicians and educators affiliated with the University of British Columbia School of Medicine. The Aboriginal Family Medicine Residency is incorporated into the Victoria site training program along with other Family Practice and Royal College residents.

The Doris and Howard Hiatt Residency in Global Health Equity and Internal Medicine

Institution: Brigham and Women's Hospital
Affiliation: Harvard University School of Medicine
Location: Boston, Massachusetts
Year Established: 2003
Disciplines: Internal Medicine and Medicine-Pediatrics
Enrollment: 6 residents per year
Website: www.brighamandwomens.org/socialmedicine/gheresidency.aspx

Brief Overview and History
The Doris and Howard Hiatt Residency in Global Health Equity and Internal Medicine is a four-year program that leads to eligibility for certification by the American Board of Internal Medicine (ABIM.) Potential applicants must first apply to the Internal Medicine Residency at Brigham and Women's Hospital. Accepted applicants may then submit an application to the Global Health Equity Residency in November of their first year of residency training. Most residents elect to earn an MPH from the Harvard School of Public Health during their residency, with tuition covered by the program. The program has strong links to domestic and overseas sites, staffed throughout the year by several faculty as well as host country clinicians. The primary emphasis is on clinical care, providing residents a chance to develop excellent clinical skills as well as those relating to health advocacy and program management. Program emphasis is on promoting social equity and on getting residents to think more broadly about what global health means, domestically and internationally.

Program Goals and Objectives
The combined residency training program in global health equity and internal medicine seeks to:

- Provide clinical training in internal medicine both domestically and abroad
- Prepare physicians to address the impact of economic, societal, political, and adverse environmental factors on health status
- Develop quantitative skills in public health, including clinical epidemiology, biostatistics, decision sciences, and health services research;
- Train future leaders in global/domestic health program administration and advocacy, effecting policy change, coalition building and procurement of funding; and,
- Provide mentorship to trainees seeking applied and/or research careers in addressing health disparities.

Curriculum Highlights and Notable Rotations

Global Health Equity residents complete a total of 48 months of multidisciplinary training including 3 years directly relevant to the subject. This expanded program fulfills the requirements for Internal Medicine board certification, as well as for an MPH while incorporating training and education in global health equity.

The PGY2 year includes a program orientation consisting of a group trip to a field site, one week of class instruction and 2 months of required rotations in Africa. In the PGY 3 and 4, residents engage in 3 months of MPH instruction and 2-3 months at a field site each year.

The program of study and field training include the following:

- Clinical training in internal medicine, including an ambulatory continuity clinic that is culturally competent and promotes reduction of health disparities.
- Overseas or domestic field work, research and coursework. All residents complete a project in one of three areas: a clinical research paper; a project leading to improvement in clinical services in their field site; or, an evidence-based policy recommendations paper, preferably with publication. The MPH program has specific project requirements.
- Preparation in addressing the impact of economic, societal, political and adverse environmental factors on health status.
- Mentorship in clinical medicine and health disparities service and research.
- Graduate coursework leading to an MPH at the Harvard School of Public Health.
- Didactic seminars in global health equity.
- Longitudinal research in conjunction with Division of Global Health Equity faculty.

Over the three program years, residents spend most or all of 14 months at field sites, reduced by 6 months if they matriculate in the MPH program. Residents may choose from among the following field sites that have been developed over the years by the Division of Global Health Equity and Partners In Health, a Boston-based NGO.

- *Zanmi La Santé*: serving a population of 500,000 in rural Haiti
- *Socios En Salud*: providing TB-related and primary care services in Lima, Peru
- *Partners In Health Russia*: providing TB-related services in Siberia, Russia

- *The Prevention and Access to Care and Treatment (PACT) Project*: providing HIV-related health promotion and harm reduction services in Boston
- *Equipo de Apoyo en Salud y Educación Comunitaria:* providing outpatient care to indigenous people in Chiapas, Mexico
- *Inshuti Mu Buzima:* providing services related to HIV, TB and malaria in Rwinkwavu, Rwanda
- *Bo-Mphato Litsebeletsong tsa Bophelo:* providing care to HIV and TB patients and women's health at multiple locations in Lesotho
- *Abwenzi Pa Za Umoyo*: treating HIV/AIDS patients and training community health workers in the southwestern corner of Malawi
- *Indian Health Service*: providing clinical services at sites in Navajo Nation

Faculty
The program has a field-based faculty member at each clinical site overseas, as well as two mostly Boston–based faculty within the Division of Global Health Equity in the BWH Department of Medicine.

Enhanced Skills Program in Global Health & the Care of Vulnerable Populations

Institution/Affiliation: University of Toronto School of Medicine
Location: Toronto, Ontario, Canada and affiliated sites
Disciplines: Family Medicine
Enrollment: 2 PGY3 residents per year
Website:
http://www.dfcm.utoronto.ca/prospectivelearners/prosres/pgy3.htm

Brief Overview and History
The one-year Enhanced Skills Program in Global Health at the University of Toronto Medical School recognizes that primary health care is the foundation of equitable access to health,[1] and the central role which family medicine plays in primary health care.[2] The program benefits from the experience of the Department of Family and Community Medicine at the University of Toronto in collaborative capacity building in primary care overseas. The program seeks to train primary care physician leaders in work with underserved communities defined beyond geographical boundaries. It utilizes international clinical experience, and harnesses benefits not only for learners but for the local community, including the enhanced recruitment of students into family medicine, the enhanced selection of rural practice sites after graduation and improved cultural competency.[3]

Program Goals and Objectives
The program strives to enhance the ability of Canadian family physicians to competently address global health issues both locally and abroad. The training program objectives include:

1.   To enhance the skills and knowledge of family physicians in the areas relevant to global health to enable them to work more effectively in low-resource settings in Canada and abroad.
2.   To foster the development of collaborative relationships to support primary health care in low-resource settings locally, nationally and internationally
3.   To assist the development of networks and resources to support the work of family physicians in global health locally and abroad.
4.   To set the foundations of a Master's degree in global health for clinicians

Curriculum Highlights and Notable Rotations

- The curriculum begins with a one month introductory course on international health at the University of Arizona.
- Following the introduction course, residents spend four months at the University of Toronto pursuing didactic training in graduate

courses which include Teaching and Learning in the Health Professions. During this time, residents also perform clinical work in longitudinal electives.

- The final six months of the year are spent working on clinical and capacity building projects at a partner site, which include St-Gabriel Hospital in Namitete, Malawi and Howard Hospital in Zimbabwe.
- Evaluation is based on resident portfolio: geo-journal, rotation evaluations, teaching and learning evaluation, self-reflective dossier, practicum report, scholarly contribution.

Faculty

Teaching faculty include University of Toronto physicians and educators, as well as faculty at the University of Arizona (for the introductory month) and partner site faculty for the extended rotation in the second half of the year.

International Health Track at the Rainbow Center for Global Child Health

Institution: University Hospitals Case Medical Center-Rainbow Babies and Children's Hospital
Affiliation: Case Western Reserve University School of Medicine
Location: Cleveland, Ohio
Year established: 1987
Disciplines: Pediatric Residents & Internal Medicine/Pediatrics residents
Enrollment: 4 residents per year
Website:
http://www.uhhospitals.org/rainbowchildren/tabid/642/Default.aspx

Brief Overview and History
The IH Program at Rainbow Babies and Children's Hospital was established by Dr. Karen Olness in 1987. To date, Rainbow IH Program residents have completed electives in 32 countries on 4 continents and have received scholarships and awards from local and national organizations.

Program Goals and Objectives

- Providing high-quality global health training for pediatric and combined internal medicine-pediatric residents
- Providing experiences to help residents develop sensitivity to health care disparities and their causes.
- Provide experiences in child health epidemiology and public health.
- Providing clinical experiences to help residents improve skills in cross cultural pediatrics in the United States.
- Continually improving an innovative, nationally recognized model for resident education in global health.

Curriculum Highlights and Notable Rotations
The aim of the Rainbow International Health Program is to include a component of global health teaching to any Pediatric or Medicine-Pediatric trainee who is inclined to join the track. Highlights include:

- Monthly lecture series: The IH Program has a curriculum with lectures throughout the year. Topics include infectious diseases, epidemiology, nutrition, neonatal care, humanitarian emergencies, international research, the role and impact of NGOs, ethical issues and others. The IH lecture series are integrated within the residency program and all residents are encouraged to attend.
- Journal Clubs: There are 4 journal clubs per year.

- Electives: A defined and pre-approved 4-6 weeks project with pre-elective preparation and post-elective reports.
- Faculty Mentoring: The program has a core of International Health faculty, as well as additional mentors in Family Medicine and Behavioral and Developmental Pediatrics, with extensive experience abroad who participate in mentoring the residents.
- Presentations: Residents present their experience at the Annual IH Grand Rounds in May of each academic year. Some residents have presented their projects and/or research at national conferences.
- Course: "Management of Humanitarian Emergencies: Focus on Children and Families". This unique and intense week-long course is recommended to IH junior and senior residents interested in pediatric disaster response – 40 hours total.
- Joining faculty in unanticipated opportunities. Residents have had the opportunity to join faculty traveling to disaster-affected areas. Most recently, two graduating senior residents have traveled to Haiti as part of a medical team during the recent earthquake.

Faculty
Includes a Director of the International Health Program and one full- time administrator. Teaching faculty are primarily from Case Western Reserve Medical School. Faculty also include volunteer educators at international rotation sites for residents who choose to pursue visiting rotations. In addition, one of the Pediatric Chief Residents is appointed the task of coordinating and blending the IH track into the Pediatric Education Curriculum.

Johns Hopkins Urban Health Medicine-Pediatrics Residency Program

Institution: Johns Hopkins University School of Medicine
Location: Baltimore, Maryland
Year Established: 2010
Disciplines: Internal Medicine-Pediatrics
Website: www.hopkinsmedicine.org/medpeds_urban_health

Brief Overview and History
With the passage of healthcare reform, the need for primary care physicians and leaders has never been more acute. The city of Baltimore, Maryland faces a primary care workforce crisis while simultaneously contending with problems prevalent in the inner-city: poverty, chronic disease, substance abuse, psychiatric illness, urban violence, literacy issues, and health care disparities.

In order to address known and anticipated health care disparities, the Johns Hopkins Departments of Internal Medicine and Pediatrics provide an innovative urban health (UH) residency program. This combined internal medicine and pediatrics UH residency program trains primary care physician leaders to provide effective, longitudinal, comprehensive, coordinated, patient-centered care for the vulnerable, underserved inner-city patient and who will serve as systems-level change agents and advocates.

Program Goals and Objectives
The dual certification in internal medicine and pediatrics will prepare graduates to care comprehensively for patients of all ages throughout the entire life cycle and address health disparities in our community. The UH residency program will create primary care physicians who can effectively care for patients and families in Baltimore in collaboration with other health care professionals. As has been true for all of The Johns Hopkins Hospital housestaff training programs, it is anticipated that these physicians will become the future leaders of urban primary care on a local, state, and national level.

Curriculum Highlights and Notable Rotations
The unique UH curriculum will couple traditional internal medicine-pediatrics requirements with expanded training in the health issues that burden urban settings such as psychiatric illness, urban violence, substance abuse, HIV/AIDS care, prison health, and disparities. The program will provide learning experiences in cost-effective care, quality improvement, patient safety, evidence-based practice, medical informatics, health care financing, ethics, end-of-life care, and practice management.

The UH clinic is housed in the East Baltimore Medical Center which is located in the Greenmount East neighborhood, a Health Professional Shortage Area (HPSA). A Patient-Centered Medical Home, the clinic will also feature inter-professional training as residents and nurse practitioner students will care for patients together.

After four years of combined internal medicine-pediatrics training, the graduates will pursue a two-year tuition-free master's degree in public health, health science, education, or business with an emphasis on urban health issues while providing ambulatory care in a HPSA designated clinic.

The UH curriculum is a unique feature of this training program and includes the following topics:

- Substance Abuse Rotation: Residents will participate in an intensive 4-week rotation and a longitudinal experience of at least six months, enabling residents to observe the long-term trials and tribulations of substance abuse.

- Psychiatry Experiences: A 4-week rotation and longitudinal experience coordinated by Johns Hopkins Psychiatry that provides enhanced psychiatry education emphasizing diagnosis of major psychiatric illnesses, outpatient treatment of major depression, and identification of patients with dual diagnoses.

- Urban Violence Rotation: Residents will perform domestic violence/sexual assault evaluations for children and adults, analyze the impact of domestic violence while providing collaborative medical care at the House of Ruth School of Nursing clinic, learn to recognize and evaluate child abuse, and attend the monthly police department domestic violence autopsy conference.

- HIV Care: Residents will care for pediatric and adult patients infected with HIV in an outpatient setting.

- Urban Health Institute Partnership: Residents will learn methods to both minimize barriers to care and maximize care opportunities, partner with community health workers to provide in-home interventions, and forge bonds with the community by meeting leaders and participating in outreach.

- Prison Medicine Rotation

- Baltimore City Health Department: Residents will spend one month at the BCHD learning about the scope of clinical services, observing and participating in programs, and contributing to policy and program development.

- Communication and Cultural Competency Curriculum: Drawing on two Hopkins medical communication experts, Drs. Lisa Cooper (MacArthur genius grant awardee) and Mary Catherine Beach, the program is developing a curriculum that will span the entire residency, focusing on motivational interviewing and effective cross-cultural communication, fostering cultural competence.

Faculty

Teaching faculty draw from the Johns Hopkins University Department of Internal Medicine and the Department of Pediatrics, as well as from the larger faculty of the Johns Hopkins School of Medicine.

Lawrence Family Medicine Residency

Insitution: Greater Lawrence Family Health Center
Affiliation: Lawrence General Hospital
Location: Lawrence, Massachusetts
Year Established: 1994
Disciplines: Family Medicine
Enrollment: 8-10 residents per year
Website: http://www.lawrencefmr.org

Brief Overview and History
The family medicine residency in Lawrence, Massachusetts has many
unique aspects, including its distinction as the first accredited community
health center-sponsored residency in the United States. The program
provides care to a diverse population of patients and prides itself on its
integral role within the community, its collaborative community
partnerships, and its foundation of cultural competency. The Lawrence
residency program demonstrates that global health education and training
occurs both in one's home community as well as in international training
sites.

Program Goals and Objectives
Lawrence Family Medicine Residency is dedicated to training culturally
competent family physicians, capable of providing comprehensive primary
care to underserved communities. The program has a strong commitment to
global health programming, which reflects the predominantly Latino patient
population it serves in northeastern Massachusetts. In addition to providing
highly-regarded, full-spectrum family medicine training, the Lawrence
residency includes language and cultural immersion programs during
internship, continuous cultural and language support and education
throughout residency, and training in social determinates of health both at
the home community training site as well as at international partner sites.

Curriculum Highlights and Notable Rotations

- 10-day intensive Spanish language course at Dartmouth College
  for all 1st year residents prior to beginning clinical training.
- Residents train at Greater Lawrence Family Health Center (a
  community-based clinic) and Lawrence General Hospital,
  providing care for a diverse, underserved patient population in
  Lawrence, Massachusetts (30 minutes north of Boston.)
- Several global health lectures are given per year in the core
  curriculum, provided by both faculty and residents with global
  health experience.
- 1st year residents participate in a week-long visit to sister program
  in Dominican Republic for educational and cultural exchange.

- The residency program accommodates the training goals of many residents by allowing flexible scheduling to complete additional field work or complementary degrees (e.g., MPH).
- Protected time for extramural rotations includes 1 week during intern year in the Dominican Republic, and up 2 consecutive months during 3rd year elective time.
- Established partner sites in Nicaragua and the Dominican Republic.
- Longstanding relationship with the non-governmental organization Bridges to Community, a partner in improving public health access in underserved communities in Nicaragua.
- Structured, longitudinal relationship and elective with Nicaraguan clinical site, including pre-departure preparation and structured mentoring.

Faculty
A multicultural group of faculty with diverse interests supports resident education and training at the Lawrence Family Medicine Residency. Many Lawrence faculty have previously worked in clinical and research positions in underserved communities both in the United States and abroad. Several faculty members have substantial global health experience and act as mentors.

Montefiore Residency Program in Social Medicine

Insitution: Montefiore Medical Center
Affiliation: Albert Einstein College of Medicine
Location: Bronx, New York
Year Established: 1970
Disciplines: Family Medicine, Internal Medicine, Pediatrics
Enrollment: 10 residents per year
Website: http://www.montefiore.org/prof/departments/family/rpsm/

Brief Overview and History
The purpose of the programs in Social Internal Medicine (SM, since 1970) and Primary Care (PC, since 1976), now the Residency Program in Primary Care and Social Internal Medicine (PC/SM) at Montefiore is to produce, in an academic environment of innovation and commitment, clinicians and physicians leaders who are equipped to improve the health of society, particularly among underserved populations domestically and globally. The PC/SM curriculum in global health is a natural outgrowth of Montefiore's nationally recognized focus on achieving health through social justice and confronting health disparities. It encompasses a set of courses, rounds, and experiential opportunities within the broader residency curriculum, combined with an intense field experience in a district hospital in Uganda. While all residents in the PC/SM Programs are eligible for the global health opportunities described below (and 90% participate), many categorical and family medicine residents join as well.

Program Goals and Objectives
The goals of the Global Health Curriculum are to develop outstanding clinical skills that can be applied in diverse resource-poor settings in both the developing and developed world; To provide both the intellectual and the experiential foundations of culturally competent clinical practice; To better prepare residents for roles as health care leaders by presenting an inclusive global vision of the biological and social determinants of health; To illustrate and appreciate health disparities in their broadest context and the synergy between domestic and global inequity; To develop skills in population-based research and community-oriented primary care that can be employed to effect social change and improve society's health.

Curriculum Highlights and Notable Rotations
The Montefiore program leads to Board eligibility in Internal Medicine in 3 years, the amount of time residents spend abroad in their training is limited to 2 months, most residents spending one. However, global health themes and domestic global health experiences run throughout the home-based curriculum. Completion of the 3-year PC/SM Residency earns credits towards an MPH at Einstein College of Medicine (Einstein).

Of the 33 months of residency training, residents spend 16 on inpatient general and subspecialty wards and in intensive care units; 12 months in General

Medicine (GM) rotations; and 5 elective months. The GM months, which distinguish the PC/SM Program, incorporate ambulatory medicine practice in our South Bronx community health center (Comprehensive Health Care Center), in the poorest urban congressional district in the country with a largely immigrant population, with a special academic focus that varies each month. Prominently emphasized themes include: Clinical Epidemiology and Health Systems Research, Community Medicine, Global Health, Immigrant Health, Women's Health, HIV-AIDS, Human Rights, Substance Abuse, Geriatrics, and Behavioral Medicine.

The global health curriculum incorporates both local (domestic) and international global health into its 3 year curriculum.

Local global health opportunities include:

- **OPEN-IT Clinic and Immigrant Health Rounds:** (Opportunities Pro-immigrant and Newcomer International Travel). Resident-trained Community Health Workers link recent immigrants with health care through the bimonthly OPEN-IT Clinic. After each OPEN-IT Clinic, 1-hour rounds focus on the diseases, health systems, economics, politics, and cultures of the countries of origin of the patients seen the OPEN-IT Clinic.
- **The Human Rights Clinic** of the Montefiore PC/SM Program: Started through collaboration between the Montefiore PC/SM Program and Doctors of the World in 1987, this monthly clinic was one of the first in the nation -- and the only whose providers are residents -- to document international torture and care for its victims.

International global health rotations include:

- **Health, Human Rights and Liberation Medicine:** an eight seminar course offered during the October GM Month that explores health and human rights both nationally and internationally.
- **Global Health Course:** This very highly rated course, offered at the end of the PGYII is an intense immersion into the clinical, social, economic, and political realities of health in the developing world. It features over 100 hours of seminars led by globally involved faculty from the Einstein, the Columbia University School of Public Health, and multiple NGOs. The course is a prerequisite for the field experiences described below.
- **Uganda, GH Field Experience:** In collaboration with Doctors for Global Health and Einstein, the PC/SM Program has developed a close relationship with a rural hospital and district in southwest Uganda, in Kisoro. PGY3 residents can elect to work for one month caring for patients of a severely understaffed district hospital. For many, the experience has transformed their career

direction and sense of themselves as physicians. A second month can be elected as a research option (see below).

- GH Research option: For residents who have global health experience before residency, are likely to pursue a career in global health, and apply to the PC/SM Program stating their desire to get involved with global health research during residency, a second month abroad can be elected in clinical research. This research is carried out under faculty supervision and can take place either in Uganda or in another site in the developing world. The entire project is not expected to be completed during that one-month field experience but rather the field work is but one part of a multi-component project whose conceptualization, Institutional Review Board application, analysis, and manuscript preparation occur in New York.

A word about the field experience in Uganda: The PC/SM Residency Program is committed to serving underserved populations in the Bronx and abroad and to capacity building in areas of need. Despite the wealth of international opportunities available through the work of Einstein/Montefiore faculty involved globally, the program has chosen to stay with and contribute to *one* site in Kisoro, Uganda. In this way, through the contributions of its residents, Montefiore's PC/SM program is able to provide this understaffed rural facility with consistent staffing every month, organize an ambitious continuing medical education series for its staff, and contribute to its Village Health Worker Program. The experience has been universally acclaimed by those who have participated, and in the context of a 3-year residency, has clearly met its stated educational goals.

Faculty

At present (2010-2011), the program has three core GH faculty, each of whom devotes 25%-50% time to global health curriculum and field activities. Beyond the residency program per se, there is a wide range of global health-oriented faculty who are members of the Global Health Center at Einstein. Einstein has a 30-year history of involvement in global health research, education, and capacity-building, now represented by 30 to 40 faculty members with international research and service projects - an extensive network of available mentors.

Women and Newborns –Didactic, Outreach, Opportunities and Research (WONDOOR)

Institution: University Hospitals Case Medical Center, MacDonald Women's Hospital
Academic Affiliation: Case Western Reserve University School of Medicine
Location: Cleveland, Ohio
Year Established: 2004
Disciplines: Obstetrics and Gynecology
Enrollment: 2 residents per year
Website:
http://www.uhhospitals.org/HealthProfessionals/WONDOORGlobalHealth Program/tabid/7698/Default.aspx

Brief Overview and History
W.O.N.D.O.O.R (pronounced "one door") *Wo*men and *N*ewborns –*D*idactic, *O*utreach, *O*pportunities *and Research* is a new and innovative global health program that grew out of the concept that women should have the same opportunity to enter the same door to quality health care whether they are living abroad or in our own communities. The following principles are the core challenges that are fundamental to the success of this program:

- Need for more personnel able to address global health problems
- Strong resident and student interest in global health issues and experiences
- Insufficient qualified faculty.
- Limited appropriate teaching materials
- Global International health education can affect career choices
- Health education can enhance the ability to work in cross-cultural settings.
- Global health education can better prepare residents to serve the communities in which they are placed

The residency trainee program at MacDonald Women's Hospital has offered a short international experience to our residents over the past six years. The recognition and respect for a comprehensive global health program that is sustainable and impacts the overall wellbeing of women while training young physicians is the forward thinking at University Hospitals. This vision will enrich our unique program. Care of women globally is currently the hallmark of only three other residency training programs in this country.

Program Goals and Objectives

The disparity between developed countries and developing countries as it relates to maternal and child morbidity and mortality continues to plague the Millennium Goals as outlined in 2002. Women continue to succumb to deaths from preventable causes. These causes are hemorrhage, infection, pre-eclampsia and induced abortion. The most recent statistics noted by the World Health Organization notes the maternal mortality in developed countries versus developing countries to be 1/4000 and 1/17 respectively. In 2000, there were 6.3 million neonatal deaths worldwide. Neonatal deaths in Africa, Asia, Caribbean and Latin America are 62/1000, 50/1000, 31/1000 and 20/1000, respectively (WHO 2010). These statistics continue to drive the agenda to prepare physicians to be global providers.

The overall objective of the program is consistent with the United States global health initiative focused on achieving the WHO Millennium Development Goals of improving maternal and child health. The faculty at MacDonald Women's hospital believes that investment in training residents, faculty, nurses and students as global health providers will significantly contribute to this effort. A multi-specialty advisory board is actively involved in the global health program as mentors and educators. Local and international collaborations offer participants experiences locally and travel abroad to sharpen their clinical skills in under- resourced environments. These collaborations will potentially establish sustainable programs with the hope of positive measurable outcomes.

The program enhances obstetric and gynecology education curriculum and acquisition of a broader skill base by providing comprehensive clinical and research opportunities – ultimately promoting careers in global health while establishing programs that promote quality of life for women is our mission.

Specific objectives of the W.O.N.D.O.O.R program are to:

- exposes trainees to the health care challenges of women living in under resourced communities,
- improve clinical evaluation and diagnostic skills consistent with skill level
- improve operative skills,
- improve understanding of cultural practices that influence clinical competence
- Improve understanding and initiate programs in research that improve global health care.

Curriculum Highlights and Notable Rotations

The Global Health Scholars curriculum is designed to complement the MacDonald Women's/Case Western Medical Centers residency program in Obstetric & Gynecology and Reproductive Biology. Two scholars are selected per year through an application., letter of recommendation and a faculty interview.

This three year program seeks to meet outlined objectives through:

- Required didactic sessions
- Independent reading with written reflective summaries that propose thoughtful   solutions to various challenges
- Off –site journal club to include interested residents and faculty
- Attendance and/or presentation at one international conference during the PGY-1 & PGY-2 years.
- Clinical rotation (12 weeks) at a local clinic serving immigrants, refugee or homeless women
- Four weeks of international travel during the PGY-3 and/or PGY-4 years to a developing country focusing on a selected women's health issue.
- One grand rounds presentation focusing on international health care during the PGY-3 year
- Completion of outlined competencies evaluated via written or oral testing and demonstration of mastered clinical skills
- A final project that outlines a current international women's health care challenge that is a potential publishable document.
- Participants are required to meet with their assigned mentors and the global health director quarterly.
- A self-evaluation which includes professional objectives and a program evaluation is required at the end of each academic year. These completed documents must be submitted prior to the annual meeting with the director. All individual meetings must be completed prior to the July didactic session.

Unique rotations in the curriculum include:

- Short term international experience: PGY-3 or PGY-4 residents may travel during their third year research block if the time period is approved by the resident director. A minimum of four weeks is required by both our institution and the hosting institution. The Global Health Program will assist all residents in securing an appropriate international mentor(s) and will act as an advocate to insure development of a reciprocal training and educational relationship with the host institution. Fourth year medical students and nurses may also travel with residents and faculty mentors. Current international partners are Georgetown Public Hospital/University of Guyana Medical School, Guyana, and the Robert Fitkin Memorial Hospital/University of Swaziland, Swaziland, and Africa. Senegal and Sierra Leone are potential upcoming sites.

- Research exposure: an option for all participants at established collaborative research sites.

Global Health Fellowship in Obstetrics and Gynecology
The development and implementation of a Fellowship in Global Health is well underway. This two year post-graduate program will be available for applicants beginning in July of 2012. Didactics will be completed at Case Western Reserve University with concurrent experiences at local immigrant and refugee clinics. The fellow will spend approximately 18 months in under-resourced communities concentrating on program strategies that impact the health care of women.

University of California San Francisco Global Health Clinical Scholars Program

Institution: University of California San Francisco
Location: San Francisco, California
Year Established: 2006
Disciplines: Current medical and surgical residents, trainees in nursing, dentistry, pharmacy and public health at UCSF
Enrollment: a yearly cohort of 24 scholars
Website: www.globalhealthsciences.ucsf.edu/education/ClinicalScholars

Brief Overview and History
The University of California, San Francisco Global Health Clinical Scholars Program was established in 2006. It is one of a number of programs that make up the UCSF Pathway to Discovery in Global Health, which spans medical school to fellowships, and includes the first master's degree program in global health in the United States. The Global Health Clinical Scholars Program continues to be the most broadly multidisciplinary resident global health programs in the country. To date the program has had participants from 12 different medical school residencies: orthopedic surgery, radiology, psychiatry, neurology, OB/GYN, urology, anesthesia, general surgery, dermatology, medicine, family and community medicine, and pediatrics. The program originally included 16 residents, and has expanded to 24 per year. It also includes residents from UCSF pharmacy and dentistry schools and graduate level nursing students.

Program Goals and Objectives
The UCSF Global Health Clinical Scholars Program seeks to:

- Develop a cohort of scholars from different specialties with similar interests in global health
- Teach basic global health principles through a range of fundamental topics
- Increase networking opportunities with global health faculty
- Provide exposure to multiple career paths within global health
- Foster interdisciplinary scholarly work in global health within UCSF clinical training programs
- Encourage a commitment to global health issues

Curriculum Highlights and Notable Rotations

- Three-week Intensive Course in Global Health: scholars participate in didactic and small group sessions with leaders in global health to discuss a variety of global health topics, and learn basic research and program evaluation skills. This course explores areas that are not specific to any one discipline, like economics, politics, ethnography, and ethics. Issues such as work-force shortages are examined, and participants work on problems in small groups to better understand them. Although some basic topics are examined in-depth, the course is intended to provide an overview of important global health issues, the vocabulary used in various relevant disciplines, and suggest resources for further study. There is also a focus on developing and planning for a project to be complete during the rest of the time in training at UCSF.

- Monthly Global Health Network Meetings: Scholars arrange evening meetings on a monthly basis, which help foster community building among scholars. The scholars may invite guest speakers, lead journal reviews, review projects, or arrange for documentary viewings with discussions.

- Web-based Longitudinal Curriculum: Scholars review a series of global health teaching modules and may also develop their own modules over the year that focus on a range of global health topics. Some of these modules have been put on the GHEC modules project website.

- Scholarly Project: Under the mentorship of a UCSF faculty member, scholars are required to design and complete an academic project in global health that will be disseminated in one or more forums. As a basic requirement, scholars present their work at the end of each academic year at a UCSF "research festival". The project can involve clinical research, program development or evaluation, policy work, educational tool development, or other innovative inquiries at home or abroad.

- Immersion Experience: Depending on their school and program, scholars generally spend a minimum of one month in a resource-scarce country practicing clinical medicine, conducting a research project, or participating in program development. To ensure that our programs are mutually beneficial, we encourage scholars to go to sites where UCSF has longitudinal projects (such as Kisumu, Kenya; Kampala, Uganda; and Muhimbili, Tanzania), facilitating a rich commitment to truly collaborative research and capacity building.

Faculty
UCSF clinical faculty, faculty from other UC institutions including UC Berkeley, and regional and international scholars participate in both the intensive three week didactic course, as well as the longitudinal curriculum. Advisors to scholars are generally from the faculty of the UCSF School of Medicine, but may include professionals at collaborating institutions.

University of Pennsylvania Graduate Medical Education Global Track for Residents

Institution: University of Pennsylvania School of Medicine
Location: Philadelphia, Pennsylvania
Year Established: 2006
Disciplines: Internal medicine, partial participation for residents in other disciplines
Enrollment: 4 internal medicine residents per year, 1-2 additional residents in other programs
Website:
http://www.med.upenn.edu/globalhealth/UPENNSOMGlobalHealthPrograms-GME

Brief Overview and History
In 2006, the University of Pennsylvania School of Medicine joined a four school consortium of newly developing global health curricula. In 2008, the Department of Medicine at PennMed launched a track in global health for interested residents. Major elements in the track are: international rotations in developing countries; continuity clinics in Philadelphia for medically underserved populations; a one-month intensive seminar program; bi-weekly on-line curriculum on relevant topics; monthly speakers and discussions and a scholarly project pertinent to global health. Some components of the track are also available to residents in other specialties. The program has a strong foundation with its primary partner institution, Princess Marina Hospital in Gaborone, Botswana. Plans are underway to expand this program to incorporate other rich international health experiences. The program also includes instruction in a basic global health curriculum, mentorship, support for scholarly activities and interaction with the broader global health community.

Program Goals and Objectives
The overarching objective of the University of Pennsylvania program is to help nurture and train future global health professionals while simultaneously helping to improve health care training in partner countries. The global health residency track has several goals:

- To provide educational opportunities that will nurture and train health professionals who want to address health disparities, domestically or internationally.
- To promote physician advocacy and service through working with our community and global partners to improve health care and medical education.
- To expose participants to public health and population-based approaches to prevention and care in under-resourced settings.

Curriculum Highlights and Notable Rotations

Residents will participate in a month-long course in global health featuring lecturers from the Penn community as well as from the broader global health community. Longitudinal curriculum includes:

- Journal clubs lead by global health program residents
- Web-based curriculum including cases focusing on tropical and neglected disease, and case studies and questions about current policy issues in global health

Each resident will spend a minimum of six weeks in abroad in their PGY3 year and between 6 weeks abroad in the PGY2 year.

- Botswana: Resident responsibilities will include direct clinical care of patients in Princess Marina Hospital, a busy public hospital in the capital, Gaborone. Residents will be expected to help with intern education and supervision. A major goal of the Penn-Botswana partnership is to build sustainable, quality health education and work with health providers and the government of Botswana to strengthen health care at Princess Marina Hospital.
- Kenya: Residents will work at Mbagathi District Hospital, the public district hospital for Nairobi with experiences offered in both inpatient medicine and outpatient HIV clinic. Residents will also have the opportunity to work with local Kenyan NGOs to investigate public health questions pertaining to health system development and health workforce. Several projects are underway through the World Health Organization and residents will have the opportunity to work on these projects.
- Guatemala: Residents will work at the Hospitalito Atitlan in Santiago Atitlan to provide clinical care and health education to the local population. The Hospitalito is a small private facility that provides outpatient, inpatient and emergency care to residents of the surrounding region. As most patients are impoverished, care is provided on a sliding scale and in some cases, free.
- Dominican Republic (2 sites): Residents will work at the Centro de Salud in Consuelo, a small town an hour east of the capital. Residents will work with attendings to provide clinical outpatient general medical care to the Consuelo population. Additionally, residents will work with the direct of the mobile outreach medical program to travel to the surrounding sugar cane fields to provide regular continuity care to the sugar cane workers and their families. Residents will also work at CEPROSH, a full-service HIV care and treatment center in the city of Puerto Plata. Residents will work with attendings to provide clinical care to people living with HIV and will also go on outreach visits to sugar cane field sites on the border of Haiti.

In addition to the resident's primary continuity clinic, global health program residents will work in a second continuity clinic site focused on issues of community health and immigrant health:

- Prevention Point Philadelphia: Providing health care at Philadelphia needle exchange sites
- Philadelphia Health Department: STI/HIV and TB clinic
- Correctional medicine: health care in the Philadelphia prison system
- Health care for the homeless
- Migrant health and immigrant health care

Residents are encouraged to complete a scholarly project under the mentorship of a Penn faculty member. This project may focus on clinical research, policy work or programmatic questions. Where appropriate, residents are supported to work closely with partner organizations outside of the University to complete these projects.

Faculty
Faculty for the GME Global Track are from multiple departments at the University of Pennsylvania School of Medicine, as well as faculty at partner sites in Botswana, Kenya, Dominican Republic and Guatemala.

Yale/Stanford Johnson & Johnson Global Health Scholars Program

Institutions: Yale University School of Medicine, Stanford University School of Medicine
Location: Established sites in Uganda, South Africa, Eritrea, Indonesia and Liberia
Year Established: 1981
Disciplines: Internal Medicine, Primary Care, Family Medicine, Internal Medicine-Pediatrics, Obstetrics and Gynecology, and Emergency Medicine
Enrollment: 40 resident and career physicians per year, residents are mainly from Yale and Stanford
Website: http://medicinc.yale.edu/intmed/globalhealthscholars

Brief Overview and History
The Yale/Stanford Johnson & Johnson Global Health Scholars Program offers international medical experiences for residents (and career physicians) who are interested in building capacity by developing partnerships of patient-centered care and models of teaching in low resource settings. The program seeks to promote mutually beneficial learning through providing care in underdeveloped areas lacking modern medical resources, as well as invaluable medical experiences that result from practicing and teaching in a new and challenging environment.

The program grew out of the Yale University International Health Program – founded in 1981 by Drs. Michele Barry and Frank Bia in an attempt to inspire a more global vision of health care in a traditional internal medicine residency program. The Yale/Johnson & Johnson Physician Scholars in International Health Program was conceived in 2001 with the goals of expanding the existing Yale IHP to physicians in residency training from leading U.S. hospitals and universities, and offering overseas opportunities to more experienced career physicians. The program is now jointly affiliated at Yale and Stanford Universities.

Program Goals and Objectives
Over 1000 residents-in-training have participated in this unique program by working and teaching in underserved areas throughout the world. These rotations offer unusual opportunities for residents to enrich their knowledge and practice of medicine in settings with few resources. A study of Yale graduates of this program confirmed that IHP physicians were more likely than their counterparts to demonstrate social concern within their clinical practices as measured by their commitment to serve poor and immigrant populations. Rotations are largely directed at clinical experiences, service and teaching, as opposed to research. Experience gained as a Yale/Stanford Johnson & Johnson Global Health Scholar will fill all or part of the requirements for certification by the American Society of Tropical Medicine and Hygiene.

Curriculum Highlights and Notable Rotations

The Yale/Stanford Johnson & Johnson Global Health Scholars Program annually selects up to 40 physicians during their residencies and career physicians for six-week rotations at one of our mentored sites outside the US. Rotations are largely directed at clinical experiences, service and teaching, as opposed to research.

Yale/Stanford Johnson & Johnson Global Health Scholars will receive, upon completion of the rotation, a travel award ranging from $3,000 - $4,000 based on their site assignment. This financial support will serve as partial reimbursement for travel and living expenses incurred during the rotation. All scholars are required to participate in program evaluation upon completion of the rotation. Established rotation sites are in Uganda, South Africa, Eritrea, Indonesia and Liberia. Planning is underway to establish a site in Central America. Certain sites provide the opportunity to take language classes, and translation is provided when necessary. Examples of three sites as follows:

- Uganda: visiting scholars work in Mulago Hospital, Kampala, a 1,500 bed hospital which is affiliated with Makerere University Faculty of Medicine. Patients are affected by a broad range of medical and infectious diseases, including HIV/AIDS, TB, malaria and tropical medicine. Clinical responsibilities include inpatient and outpatient medicine, emergency care, community outreach and home visits, and presentation of lectures and bedside teaching. English is spoken throughout Uganda, and Luganda lessons are provided to all scholars at twice weekly lunch sessions. Due to the capacity-building efforts of the Makerere University/Yale University collaboration, there are many coordinated opportunities to experience more of Uganda through outreach opportunities at St. Stephen's Hospital, Holy Family Nazareth Secondary School and other local CBOs and through trips to Gulu, Kansesero and Rwanda.

- South Africa: scholars rotate at the Church of Scotland Hospital in Tugela Ferry, KwaZuluNatal. The 355-bed hospital is 2 hours by car from Durban, and it is affiliated with Nelson R. Mandela School of Medicine. Full-time hospital staff include 8 physicians including 2-4 intern equivalent community service doctors doing preliminary-year equivalent rotations throughout the hospital. Patients display a range of infectious diseases but most prominently HIV/AIDS and TB. Clinical responsibilities include inpatient pediatric, medical, and tuberculosis wards; outpatient antiretroviral clinic (most physician-scholars spend bulk of time at this location,) and hospice which serves as step-down like facility for patients with HIV/TB co-infection and multi-system disease; emergency and casualty service as an optional rotation with possibility of overnight call; community outreach home visits to

186

rural countryside as well as mobile-clinic on department of health van; lecture opportunities to present at weekly case conference; and potential for participation in ongoing clinical research related to TB and HIV co infection.

- Indonesia: visiting scholars work at the Alam Sehat Lestari clinic in Sukadana, West Kalimantan, Borneo, where families are able to trade health care for labor on income-generating projects. The clinic is two hours from Ketapang airport, and two fulltime physicians see 25-35 complicated patients each day. If necessary, 3 beds are available for overnight hospitalization. The spectrum of disease includes malaria, tuberculosis, pertussis, diabetes, asthma, seizure disorders, psychiatric diseases - advanced stages of many common and rare diseases. Clinical responsibilities include primarily outpatient visits with complicated patients, and bedside teaching with junior Indonesian doctors. Frequent home visits are necessary for reaching mobility limited and severely ill patients. There is minimal inpatient care, at most 3 in-patients who are cared for by the nurses. Rarely there may be some night time responsibilities. Visiting scholars may participate in community outreach at meetings both for environmental protection and health promotion. Shared housing available with our Indonesian staff and other volunteers. No language requirements exist at the Indonesian site, host physicians speak English.

Faculty

Mentors at each hospital site, chosen by program directors based on personal relationships, provide supervision and guidance during the six week rotations. At times, Yale and Stanford faculty and senior career physicians are on site as well. Two internationally experienced physicians, Michele Barry at Stanford and Asghar Rastegar at Yale are program Co-Directors and are involved on a daily basis with program management. Full-time administrative coverage and support is available at Yale for the overseas mentors and the scholars. A Global Health Programs Committee at Yale, comprised of program directors, site liaison staff, faculty and chief residents meet on a regular basis.

Global Health Fellowship Programs

Global Health Fellowship in Anesthesia

Institution: Dalhousie University School of Medicine
Location: Halifax, Nova Scotia, Canada
Year Established: 2009
Discipline: Anesthesia, 1 year postgraduate fellowship
Enrollment: 1 fellow per year
Website: http://anesthesia.medicine.dal.ca/global-health/global-health-initiatives.php

Brief Overview and History
Globally, about 234 million major surgical operations are conducted each year. In some regions, anesthesia-related mortality is as high as 1 in 150 patients receiving general anesthesia. Safe surgery requires safe anesthesia, which can only be delivered if sustainable, high-quality training and resources are available.[4]

Appropriate surgical care contributes to reductions in mortality rates from traffic accidents, conflicts and natural disasters, and anesthesia is an essential component of surgical care. A lack of health professionals trained in anesthetic care can prevent much-needed surgery from happening at all or compromise the quality of surgeries that do take place.

Safe anesthesia is essential for reducing maternal and fetal mortality, which is a millennium development goal. The most common causes of maternal death worldwide are hemorrhage, hypertensive diseases and sepsis, with a smaller proportion due to obstructed labor.[5,6] The presence of a health professional skilled in anesthetic care would prevent many of these deaths as appropriate life-saving surgical interventions could be performed. Anesthesia professionals are also skilled at recognizing and providing the need for prompt and effective resuscitation to critically ill mothers and their infants.

The Dalhousie University School of Medicine Department of Anesthesia is recognized nationally and internationally as a center of clinical excellence in anesthesia care and has one of the highest ranked residency training programs in Canada. In 2009, with the support of many faculty involved in global projects, and successful partnerships with institutions in Rwanda and Ghana, the Global Health Fellowship in Anesthesia was established. Selected fellows practice and teach at the QEII Health Sciences Centre, the largest tertiary care hospital in Atlantic Canada, and at the affiliated hospitals of the National University of Rwanda.

Program Goals and Objectives
The anesthesia global health fellowship offers many opportunities to develop skills in clinical care, teaching and research in Canada and abroad. The global health fellow will learn from faculty and staff mentors who have

extensive anesthesia experience in resource-poor countries. The fellowship seeks to provide clinical and academic leadership training for a career in global health work and to provide anesthesia care in challenging environments and to establish an anesthesia training program in a developing country.

Curriculum Highlights and Notable Rotations

- Participation in two unique courses to prepare anesthesiologists for practice in resource-limited surroundings: "Anesthesia for Developing Countries" in Kampala, Uganda, and "Anesthesia in Challenging Environments" in Halifax.
- Rotation for three to four months in Rwanda as part of the Canadian Anesthesiologists' Society International Education Foundation (CASIEF) program. CASIEF is working with the National University of Rwanda to expand and strengthen its residency program in anesthesia. In February 2010, two postgraduate residents from the University of Rwanda came to Halifax for six months to train in the Department of Anesthesia. Two more Rwandan residents will arrive in February 2011.
- Provide obstetrical anesthesia care in Ghana as part of the Kybele team, to improve maternal care in Ghana. Kybele is a humanitarian organization dedicated to improving childbirth conditions worldwide through medical education partnerships.
- Practice clinical anesthesia in Halifax.
- Supervise residents from a developing country.
- Elective in an area of interest (e.g. tropical disease, health policy.)
- Preparation of an abstract and attendance at the Canadian Society for International Health's global health conference in Ottawa.

Faculty
Include mentors and clinical anesthesiologists from the Dalhousie University School of Medicine, as well as clinical and community partners from institutions in Rwanda and Ghana.

International Emergency Medicine and Health Fellowship

Institution: University of Illinois Chicago
Location: Chicago, Illinois
Year Established: 1995
Discipline: Emergency Medicine, special consideration for other disciplines (Med-Peds, Internal Medicine, etc.)
Enrollment: 1 fellow per year, two year fellowship includes an MPH
Website: http://www.uic.edu/com/er/EMProg/intlfellowship.shtml

Brief Overview and History
Begun in 1995, the UIC international emergency medicine and health fellowship trains physicians who seek to challenge and be challenged by the international community to engage in sustainable development of global humanitarian and emergency care efforts. Since its inception, the program has trained 9 fellows in its two year program.

Program Goals and Objectives
The program strives to provide an environment which supports efforts in humanitarian assistance, encourages development of further initiatives in international health and emergency care systems, and provides leadership and leadership opportunities to effectively administer such programs. Program goals include:

1. Comprehensive application of clinical emergency medicine concepts and skills in international health.
2. Understand and apply the concepts of sustainability and capacity building in international emergency medicine and health.
3. Develop the ability to assess international health systems and emergency medical care systems and identify pertinent health issues to aid in design of health programs that address identified needs.
4. Develop the knowledge to evaluate the effectiveness and quality of international health programs.
5. Establish network and skills for educational exchange, research, and funding.
6. Develop administrative skills to organize and implement emergency and/or international health programs abroad and integrate them into existing health systems.

Curriculum Highlights and Notable Rotations
Training in the fellowship will allow the fellow to tailor their experience based on individual interest while providing a foundation for work in international emergency medicine and health. Areas of focus may include EMS system development, human capacity development, disaster response, complex emergencies, relief, international public health.

The structure of the fellowship is primarily divided into six general areas:

1. <u>Clinical:</u> The fellow will work as clinical faculty in the Emergency Department at a University of Illinois teaching hospital. The fellow will be responsible for clinical work in the ED, as well as conference and grand round presentations.
2. <u>International field work:</u> The fellow will be working abroad on international health projects. These international experiences are generally arranged by the fellow with supervision of the fellowship director. These experiences can range anywhere from evaluation/research, to basic health care/intervention, to implementing new training curriculums in different countries, to disaster or public health response. It is expected that the fellow will be able to generate, at minimum, a report from each project or trip. Depending upon coursework and clinical work responsibilities, the fellow may have up to 4-5 months of international experience. The department and its fellows have partnerships both past and ongoing with:

- Pastoral de Salud, a nongovernmental organization (NGO) that provides health care in rural Guatemala
- The Chicago Medical Response Team for the Haiti earthquake disaster
- Global Emergency Care Collaborative (GECC), a non-profit organization that started an emergency department in rural Uganda and has trained Ugandan nurses to be emergency nurse practitioners.
- North Korea (DPRK) Ministry of Health to improve health delivery systems for tuberculosis and hepatitis, to build capacity of its tuberculosis national reference laboratory, and to implement mass vaccinations against Japanese encephalitis.
- Healthy Frontiers in Laos with plans to assist in emergency medicine curriculum development and training of physicians.
- FERNE, the Foundation in Education and Research in Neurologic Emergencies, a not-for-profit organization that has had involvement in Chile and South America.
- Indian NGO, Seva Mandir, on public health initiatives including developing training modules for nurses and traditional birth attendants
- Medical Teams International, doing cardiac life support training in Uzbekistan.

3. Didactic: The fellow during the course of the program will get exposure to the public health issues related to practice and international health through obtaining a masters degree in Public Health at the University of Illinois School of Public Health. The fellow will be responsible for the application to the condensed one year Professional Enhancement Program through the school. In addition, the fellow will attend courses specific to international health, including parasitology and health issues related to displaced populations.

4. Research: Each fellow is required to become involved in some aspect of a research project during the program. Collaboration is encouraged with other institutions and/or other departments. Incorporated within the research arm is exposure to grant writing and aspects of obtaining funds for projects. The research experience should include international conference attendance.

5. Administrative: The fellow will engage in administrative activity in the form of organizing, planning, and implementing different aspects of projects. The fellow will also obtain experience through programs within other institutions.

6. Language: The fellow will demonstrate efforts towards a language proficiency in a language of their choosing.

Faculty
Fellows are supported by physicians from the University of Illinois Chicago, professors from the University of Illinois School of Public Health, and on site faculty at abroad partner institutions.

The Mark Stinson Fellowship in Underserved and Global Health

Institution: Contra Costa Regional Medical Center-Family Medicine Residency
Location: Martinez, California
Year Established: 2006
Discipline: Family Medicine
Enrollment: 2-year postgraduate fellowship, one fellow per year
Website: http://www.cchealth.org/groups/stinsonfellowship

Brief Overview and History
The fluid world of theory and application in underserved/global health care demands some specialization. The Mark Stinson Fellowship seeks to prepare professionals who are self-starters and not afraid to ask the difficult questions that confront physicians seeking to provide "health for all." As an innovative program outside traditional academic confines, the program offers fellows the opportunity to explore relationships with local and remote communities on a small scale. Current ethical concerns will be a focus of study, encouraging fellows to join in debates and research on brain drain, inequities in underserved populations in the United States, the role of social justice in health care, and program funds that focus only on specific diseases such as HIV/AIDS or malaria.

Program Goals and Objectives
The Mark Stinson Fellowship in Underserved and Global Health was established to provide additional education and training to family physicians committed to the care of the underserved. The core philosophy is that underserved communities, in both the U.S.A. and abroad, share similar characteristics and have significant health care needs that must be addressed in a comprehensive fashion. The central objective of this fellowship is to produce family physicians equally adept at providing clinical and procedural services in underserved areas and leading or participating in efforts focused on sustainable changes in communities that improve the quality of life for its members.

Curriculum Highlights and Notable Rotations
The first year includes orientation and early clinical work and integration with residents, faculty, and staff at the Contra Costa Regional Medical Center. Academic coursework for Master's Degree in Public Health at UC Berkeley will begin in late August and continue for two full semesters. During this time the fellow will continue to perform approximately 8-12 hours of work in the county, either in clinical or hospital settings.

The second year of the fellowship begins after completion of coursework for the professional MPH degree. During this 12-month period, the fellow will become an integral part of the physician community in the county's health system, including outpatient clinical responsibilities of 16 hours per week. Additionally, 12 hours will be allotted for inpatient skill building, which may include time spend on labor and delivery, in the operating room, and in the intensive care units. Medical education activities are encouraged.

The remaining portion of each week during the second year is devoted to study, research, and initiation of the required project. Fellows have 2 months to pursue research and field work, including a review of current literature on underserved and global health, primary health care, and current educational efforts. The program has partnership connections to institutions and sites in Indonesia, Africa, Central and South America, the South Pacific, and Europe. Relationships have been formed with Refuge International, Global Health through Education, Training and Service, and THE NETWORK: Through Unity for Health (TUFH).

Each fellow is expected to complete a paper suitable for publication in a journal or for a high-quality presentation to either the local medical and health community or a conference audience. MPH course work and research will be put into practice by fellows during the second year, in ongoing work in either rural or urban underserved communities in California or projects in international settings. These activities are intended to foster a lifelong balance between clinical medical services and public health/academic/community development.

Faculty
Fellows are supported by Contra Costa Family Medicine Residency faculty, as well as faculty at externally linked institutions, such as UC Berkeley, UC San Francisco and the Global Health Education Consortium.

Additional Resources

Directory of Grants and Fellowships in the Global Health Sciences Grants and Fellowships for Postdoctoral Researchers
John E. Fogarty International Center, United States National Institutes of Health http://www.fic.nih.gov/funding/postdocdir.htm

Fellowships, Scholarships and Funding Listing
Johns Hopkins Center for Global Health
http://www.hopkinsglobalhealth.org/resources/funding/index.html

Fellowships in Public Health and Health Policy
Saint Louis University School of Public Health
http://publichealth.slu.edu/OSD/FellowshipsinPublicHealthandHealthPolicy.htm

N.B. For discipline specific directories of global health training (e.g. orthopedics global health fellowships) search the appropriate specialty society home page (e.g. www.aaos.org for the American Academy of Orthopedic Surgeons.)

References

[1] World health Organization. Declaration of Alma Ata. Geneva, Switz: World health organization 2006. Available from http://www.who.int/hpr/NPH/docs/declaration_almaata.pdf

[2] Health Services Research 38(3). June 2003 available at http://www.hc-sc.gc.ca/hcs-sss/prim/about-apropos/index_e.htmlearch

[3] Ramsay AH, Haq C, Gjerde CL, Rothenberg D. Career influence of an international health experience during medical school. *Fam. Med* 2004; 36(6): 412-6
-- National Residency Match Program (NRMP) 2008 at www.nrmp.org. Accessed June 2, 2010.
-- Chamberlain, J; Cull W; Melgar T; Kaelber D; Kan B. The effect of dual training in internal medicine and pediatrics on the career path and job search experience of pediatric graduates. J Pediatrics. 2007, 151:419-24.
-- NMPRA Introduction to Med-Peds Pamphlet. Accessed at http://www.medpeds.org/medpeds/NMPRApamphlet.pdf, June 2, 2010

[4] 10 Facts on Safe Surgery. World Health Organization.http://www.who.int/features/factfiles/safe_surgery/en/index.html

[5] Ronsmans C, Graham W. Maternal mortality: who, when, where and why. Lancet 2006; 368: 1189–200.

[6] Khan KS, Wojdyla D, Say L, Gulmezoglu AM, Van Look FA. WHO analysis of causes of maternal death: a systematic review. Lancet 2006; 367: 1066–74.

Kathy Pedersen

Introduction

The Global Health Education Consortium (GHEC) is a group of health professionals, educators, students, and institutions committed to improving the ability of the global workforce to meet the needs of underserved populations. One new participant in this endeavor is the physician assistant profession (PA).

The PA was developed in the United States to meet the needs of underserved communities. Given universal constraints on human resources and training, especially in underserved communities, PAs and other similar professions are gaining wider acceptance. Because the PA profession has expanded globally, it is likely that medical students and residents may work during global rotations with PAs or PA students. This section of the guidebook provides some information about the PA profession, its intersection with global health work, and the potential for collaboration with medical students, residents, and their program directors.

As public health professionals analyze the global workforce more accurately, the PA profession has emerged as one approach to addressing access issues in global health. This health worker cadre has a potential role in providing health care and expanding training capacity in the developing world. Ultimately, the skill set and training of PA-type personnel is more likely to be the near- and mid-term solution to health worker shortages in low- income areas.[1] It is useful for physicians to be aware of the strengths that PAs and other professionals bring to the global healthcare workforce.

Brief History of the PA Movement

Physicians in the United States developed the PA profession in the 1960's to provide service to rural and underserved communities. Returning Vietnam military medics and corpsmen formed the early foundation of the PA profession. Since the 1960's, the number of PAs has grown rapidly and as of 2010, clinically active PAs number more than 80,000 in the US. There are now 148 accredited PA training programs in the US, and the average training program is about 27 months long. All PAs are trained in general medical care. One former director of the Bureau of Health Professions in the US said, "Four decades into their history we are privileged to be sitting in the front row of an educational experiment that has proven enormously successful."[2] As part of the larger healthcare workforce, PAs are addressing health workforce needs in the US and globally.

Physician assistants are health care professionals licensed to practice medicine with physician supervision. PA medical education is designed to complement physician training. Within the physician-PA relationship, physician assistants exercise autonomy in medical decision-making and provide a broad range of diagnostic and therapeutic services. The PA scope of practice is determined by education and experience, state law, facility policy, and work delegation decisions made by the supervising physician. Physician assistants are also involved in education, research, and administrative services. Graduation from a PA program accredited by the Accreditation Review Commission on Education for the Physician Assistant and passage of the National Commission on Certification of Physician Assistants (NCCPA) examination are required for state licensure. To maintain national certification, practicing PAs must earn 100 hours of continuing medical education every two years and pass a recertification examination every six years. The PA profession is one of the ten fastest growing occupations in the United States.[2]

International Roots of PA Practitioners and Training

One of the greatest strengths of the PA in the global arena is adaptability to the specific health needs of other nations. While the PA profession is most developed in the United States, the concept of "an assistant or extender to the doctor" is not unique to the US. Dating back to at least the 1600's under various titles, non-physician clinicians (NPCs) exist across the globe. The Russian *feldsher*, the French *officier de santé*, and the Puerto Rican *practicante* are some examples. More current types include health extension officers (HEO), registered clinical officers (RCO), and *technicos medicos* in many countries in Latin America (See Table 1.)

Table 1: Non-Physician Clinician (NPC) Examples

Non-Physician Clinician	Country / Region
Feldshers	Russia/Eastern Europe
Officier de santé	France
Barefoot doctor	China
Community Health Technicians	Colombia, Mexico, Peru, Guyana
Registered Clinical Officer	Kenya
Practicante	Puerto Rico
Nurse Practitioner	US, Canada, UK
Medical Assistant	Ghana
Physician Extender	Haiti
Health Extension Officer	Papua New Guinea
Technicos de Medicina	Mozambique

Medic	Burma
Medex	Micronesia, Guyana
Wechekorn	Thailand
Nurse Clinician	Lesotho
Clinical Associate	South Africa

References 2, 3, 3, 4, 5, 6, 7, 8, 9

In countries with severe physician shortages, NPCs provide critically important services. For example, in some sub-Saharan African nations, the numbers of NPCs equal or exceed the numbers of physicians.[10] Hooker delineates the great variety in Sub-Saharan NPCs by title, basic entrance requirement, pre-service education, internship and scope of practice.[2] Standardization of the PA-like role is challenging. There is no current WHO category for PAs. The WHO is considering categorizing health care workers by skill set.[11]

Academic competencies and training programs for the PA-like clinician may vary by country; and the NPC and PA roles will continue to evolve. PAs are often distinguished by their physician-PA relationship. PAs exercise autonomy in medical decision-making with physician supervision. NPCs, like PAs, evolve when the health care needs and resources of the country require it, with the goal of improving access to health care and the appeal of reduced cost to the system and shorter length of professional training.

A global categorization of the many types of NPCs would need to delineate the following for each type of NPC:

- Name
- Practice location (country or region)
- Pre-service training details
- Role and area of concentration in practice
- Skill set
- Level of autonomy
- Supervision and supervisory roles
- History and evolution
- Regulation and reciprocity.

Domestic Practice in the United States

Physician Assistants are an established part of the US healthcare workforce – an efficient, flexible, accepted, adaptable, and cost-effective model for health care delivery, particularly in resource poor areas. As previously discussed, the nomenclature for PAs varies widely, including the terms:

practitioners, health care professionals, non-physician clinicians, and midlevels.

Barriers to Practice Outside the US

In addition to their domestic role, PAs practice outside the US in governmental and non-governmental organizations such as the US military, the State Department, the Peace Corps, humanitarian organizations, disaster relief agencies, and private industry. In addition to providing clinical care, PAs consult on projects and teach in academic programs outside the US. The barriers to PA practice outside the US are regulatory-based and concern appropriate supervision. There are no set standards of education, licensing, credentialing or reciprocity for PAs to work in other countries.

Ethics

The American Academy of Physician Assistants has guidelines for PAs and PA students working internationally.

> 1. PAs should establish and maintain the appropriate physician/PA team.
> 2. PAs should accurately represent their skills, training, professional credentials, identity, or service, both directly and indirectly.
>
> 3. PAs should provide only those services for which they are qualified via their training or experiences, and in accordance with all legal and regulatory processes.
>
> 4. PAs should respect the culture, values, beliefs and expectations of patients, local health care providers, and the local health care systems.
>
> 5. PAs should take responsibility for being familiar with and adhering to the customs, laws, and regulations of the country where they will be providing services.
>
> 6. When applicable, PAs should identify and train local personnel who can then assume the role of providing care and continuing the education process.[12]

These guidelines may be adapted to any setting where a resident or physician works in a team model with PA or NPC providers.

PA Involvement in Global Health Work

A large percentage of PAs have interest and involvement in overseas experiences and work. Some PA programs collaborate within their departments, medical schools, and institutions with sister institutions in other countries. Intra-academic collaboration between PA schools tends to be informal, such as shared international rotation sites between PA programs. The majority of PA programs are located in institutions/universities that have an Office of International Affairs and 32% of PA programs utilize these services.

The American Academy of Physician Assistants' (AAPA) Committee on International Affairs reports that 83 countries have expressed interest in the PA model.[13] Several PA schools in the United States work with a PA school in another country, such as the University of Kentucky with the University of Wolverhampton in England; and Arcadia University with Birmingham University in England. The University of Utah PA Program has provided distance learning to the new PA Program at the University of Queensland in Australia. The US based Physician Assistant Education Association (PAEA) developed the "International Program Development Guide" in 2004.[13] Since 2003, the AAPA has held a yearly symposium on establishment and support of international PA programs. PA leaders have attended International Medical Workforce Collaborative conferences since 2005.

In addition to providing clinical care, PA's have been active in academic medicine, advocacy and workforce organization. Recent academic highlights include a PA doctoral dissertation on the feasibility of PAs in Puerto Rico and Fulbright scholarships, including a project in Rwanda. PA leaders serve as consultants to several countries on workforce issues. In the early 1970s, PA programs were established in 15 countries, some of which exist today.[10] A global organization of PA educators started in 2008. A European organization of PAs (EUROPA) is in progress. The AAPA's PA Foundation (PAF) has funded 25 global projects in 17 countries from 2005 to 2009.

Physician Assistant consultants who help countries develop their own PA programs must make the following considerations:

- Needs assessment (identify type of health professional needed, identify stakeholders, determine feasibility for country)
- Development of an educational model
- Workforce recruitment (RN, allied health worker, IMG, CHW, post secondary school graduate, other)
- Length of program
- Cost
- Marketing to appropriate audience
- Accreditation

- Certification

Studies of United States-based PAs show that consistent interest in global health work among PA students. In a 2003 survey of PA programs, all respondents believed that international rotations benefited their students and fit into program educational philosophy. Nearly all programs reported having students who wished to participate in international rotations.[13] United States PA students working internationally are unofficial ambassadors for the benefits of Physician's Assistants to the global healthcare workforce.

According to the PAEA IAC surveys in 2007-2008, one-third of US-based PA students worked in international rotations, with the majority in Africa and the Americas. Table 2 shows common locations for international rotations, and the number of US-based PA programs with current rotations in parentheses.

Table 2: International Sites for PA rotations

Africa	*Central America/Carribean*
Ghana (5)	Belize (15)
Kenya (7)	Costa Rica (4)
South Africa (7)	Dominican Republic (4)
	Guatemala (12)
Asia	Haiti (6)
India (12)	Honduras (4)
Australia (6)	Mexico (10)
	Nicaragua (7)
Europe	
UK (9)	*South America*
	Bolivia (4)
	Ecuador (8)
	Peru (9)

For the past several years, the PAEA has conducted a survey about international activities of PA programs. Survey results in 2008 demonstrated that 99 of 145 PA programs in the US have participated in global health programs. Child Family Health International (CFHI), a US based non-profit and GHEC partner, is one organization currently assisting PA schools to arrange international student rotations.[14]

Summary

Physician assistant (PA) training was established in the United States in the late 1960's in response to physician shortage in the health care workforce. With over four decades of development, PAs have become institutionalized in American health care delivery. In 2009, there were more than 80,000 clinically active PAs in the US; and over 5,000 new PAs graduate from training programs each year. PAs are licensed by the state in which they practice, and work under a physician's supervision. The US-based PA model is young, flexible, and continues to evolve. There has been interest in and development of PA training programs internationally. Given the diverse array of non-physician clinicians (NPCs) practicing in other nations, standardization of PAs and NPCs may be difficult. The PA model may be one approach to a more equal distribution of health workers worldwide. PAs and PA-type personnel have much to offer in collaboration with physicians in the local and global arenas. GHEC and associated partners could become a valuable resource to PA training programs.

Web links

The American Academy of Physician Assistants, http://www.aapa.org
The Physician Assistant Education Association, http://www.paeaonline.org
International Medical Volunteers Association, at http://imva.org/Pages/chws.htm
World Federation for Medical Education, at http://www.wfme.org/
World Health Professions Association, at http://www.whpa.org/
World Medical Association, at http://www.wma.net

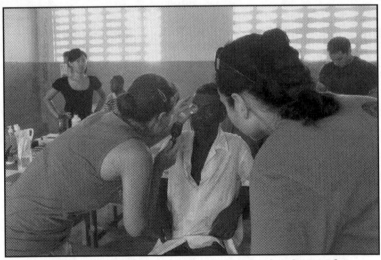

Dr. Kierstyn Napier-Dovorany demonstrating the use of an ophthalmoscope in Silegue, Haiti. (Photo credit: Irene Pulido)

References

[1] Email communication T Hall 2009.

[2] Hooker R. Cawley, J. Asprey D. Physician Assistants: Policy and Practice. Third edition. F A Davis. 2010.

[3] Strand J. The *Practicante:* Puerto Rico Physician Assistant Prototype. The Journal of Physician Assistant Education. 2006: 6 (2)

[4] Pedersen K. De Gracia D. Global Health Workforce and Physician Assistants.Global Health Education Consortium: Module 28. . http://www.globalhealth-ec.org/. 2007

[5] From International Nurse Practitioner/Advanced Practice Nurse Network, accessed at http://icn-apnetwork.org/

[6] From International Council of Nurses, accessed at http://www.icn.ch/

[7] From Lay Health Promoters website, accessed at http://community.gorge.net/ncs/background/promoters.htm

[8] From Nature and Scope of Practice of Nurse-Midwives website, http://www.icn.ch/psmidwives.thm

[9] Email communication D Smith 2002, 2008

[10] From "Non-physician clinicians in 47 sub-Saharan African countries", accessed at http://www.procor.org/discussion/displaymsg.asp?ref=3140&cate=ProCOR+Dialogue.

[11] Personal communication R Hooker 2008.

[12] Pedersen K, Hooker RS, Legler, C.Kortyna DE, Harbert K, Eisenhauer W, Baggett A. A Report on the Findings of the Ad Hoc Committee on International Physician Assistant Education. Perspectives on Physician Assistant Education 2003:14 (4)

[13] *Physician Assistant Programs: A Guide for International Program Development;* accessed at http://www.paeaonline.org (produced November 2004.)

[14] PAEA International Affairs Committee International Clinical Rotation Survey – 2007 & 2008; accessed at http://www.paeaonline.org .

-- Hooker R., Cawley J. Future Directions. Physician Assistants in American Medicine - Second edition. Churchill Livingstone. 2003. Pages 273-287.

-- *Working Together for Health: an assessment of the current crisis in the global health workforce and proposals to tackle it over the next 10 years.* The World Health Report, 2006. Accessed at http://www.who.int/whr/2006/en/

-- Additional personal communication D Pedersen 2009, and J. LoGerfo 2008.

Resources for Teaching Global Health   12

*Melanie Anspacher, Kevin Chan, Jack Chase, Thomas Hall and
    Christopher C. Stewart*

Introduction

With the rise in recognition of the importance of global health concerns,
resources for teaching and learning global health are rapidly expanding.
Within most hospital and university settings, there are individuals with
tremendous expertise and experience in global health work. In home
communities, there may be immigrants from around the world or people
who have spent significant time living in international communities. The
most valuable information may come from those without any formal
"global health" training, but instead have the volume of knowledge and
expertise that comes from living in a community and understanding its
dynamics – strengths, weaknesses, resources, and challenges. In the
absence of adequate help locally, there are a number of wonderful resources
available to teach global health. This chapter highlights some of these
resources.

      The previous chapters detail overarching approaches to building
curriculum, such as competency-based structure and ethics-based education,
as well as tools for mentoring and evaluation. Specific topics in global
health include concepts in medicine, epidemiology, biostatistics,
engineering, psychology, sociology, bench research sciences, the
humanities and more. The list of online resources at GHEC is a powerful
tool in compiling curriculum resources. Below are some of its highlights:

On-Line Global Health Curriculum

The following websites are exceptional in their volume and quality of
online lectures, modules and workshops specifically devoted to topics in
global health:

Baylor Pediatric AIDS Initiative
Excellent online HIV curriculum with cases and questions at the end of
each chapter. Accessed at http://bayloraids.org/curriculum

Global Health Education Consortium (GHEC)
GHEC is creating more than 100 peer-reviewed global health modules on
various topics in global health. The modules topics range from clinical
concepts in medicine to skills teaching for global health to determinants of
health in underserved communities. The modules are available on the
GHEC website and include PowerPoint slides (in Macromedia *Flash*

204

format) with supplementary notes, case studies, and often, an end-of-module quiz. The GHEC teaching modules can be accessed at www.globalhealthedu.org

Globalization 101.org
Articles and modules on a wide range of topics in globalization compiled by the Carnegie Endowment for International Peace. Topics include health as well as news analyses. Accessed at www.globalization101.org/issue/index

Harvard University Human Health and Environmental Change Course
An archived semester long course from the Center for Health and the Global Environment at Harvard University on the relationship between the global environment and human health. Lecture slides and videos are available at
http://chge.med.harvard.edu/programs/education/course_2007/index.html

Johns Hopkins School of Public Health
A diverse selection of open courseware from Johns Hopkins School of Public Health, ranging from genetics to injury prevention to public health preparedness. Accessed at http://ocw.jhsph.edu

National Tuberculosis Curriculum Consortium (NTCC)
Extraordinary curricular materials relevant to TB for educators and healthcare professionals worldwide. Accessed at http://ntcc.ucsd.edu/

OpenCourseWare Consortium
The massive archive of high-quality educational materials, such as university-level courses, provided by a worldwide group of hundreds of universities and organizations devoted to expanding access to education and training. Courses may be searched by topic, language, and institution of origin. Available at www.ocwconsortium.org

Partners in Health (PIH) Model Online
Electronic versions of PIH curricula which include community public health worker (*accompagnateur*) training, guidelines for HIV and TB treatment, and discussions of nutrition, electronic medical records and equipment procurement in under-resourced communities. Accessed at
http://model.pih.org/model

Tufts Open CourseWare
Online curriculum from classes at Tufts University Graduate Schools, including the Schools of Medicine, Dentistry Nutrition, Arts and Sciences, and Public Health. Links to Tufts' resources including multilingual patient educational materials, primary and secondary education tools, information resources in statistics, social engagement and water engineering and safety. Accessed at http://ocw.tufts.edu/courses/1/CourseHome.

University of Michigan Open Educational Resources
A partnership between the University of Michigan Medical School, the
University of Michigan Library system and School of Information to
provide a hub for open source educational materials and projects, including
courses, videos, lectures and more. Find a wealth of information at
https://open.umich.edu/

University of North Carolina Gillings School of Global Public Health
UNC's Gillings School offers distance certificate programs in community
preparedness and disaster management, core public health concepts, field
epidemiology, global health, maternal child health leadership and public
health leadership. Additionally, the school website has multiple web
seminars to view on diverse topics in public and global health. Accessed at
http://www.sph.unc.edu

University of North Carolina "Nutrition in Medicine" series
An impressive high-end web-based teaching module with Flash
macromedia and includes audio, streaming video, interactive quizzes and
drop-down windows. Accessed at www.med.unc.edu/nutr/nim

*University of Pittsburgh Supercourse – Epidemiology, the Internet and
Global Health*
An online resource of 4200+ lectures in 31 languages on topics in public
health and prevention. Accessed at www.pitt.edu/~super1

USAID
A series of 41 online courses developed by the USAID Bureau of Global
Health. Each module is designed to take one to two hours to complete and
topics range from clinical topics to program organization, evaluation and
management. Free to all learners, requires creation of a username and
password. www.globalhealthlearning.org

Global Studies Resources

The following collection of links compliments the above online modules
with resources, graphs, maps and lectures on topics in globalization,
statistics and information technology:

Gapminder
An interactive site which allows the user to explore a wide array of
statistical information on major global development trends in graphical
format. Accessed at www.gapminder.org

Global Poverty Mapping Project

Includes the ability to overlay poverty maps with geographical features, agro-ecological zones, education, accessibility and services. A powerful resource for better understanding of possible causes of poverty, for better targeting of resources, and for raising donor awareness of financing needs. Accessed at www.ciesin.columbia.edu/povmap/index.html

United Nations Millennium Development Goal Indicators
The official data, definitions, methodologies and sources of the UN's Millennium Development Goals, updated frequently with current statistics and documents. Found at
http://millenniumindicators.un.org/unsd/mdg/default.aspx

Population Reference Bureau (PRB)
An excellent source of population-related data relevant to global health, including tables, graphs and slides. Learn more at
www.prb.org/datafinder.aspx

Source
Strengthening the management, use and impact of information on health and disability worldwide. The Source resource library provides selected and reviewed resources, books, reports, websites, organizations, newsletters and more. Discover more at www.asksource.info

TED Lecture Series – Ideas Worth Spreading
The online archive of over 700 thought-provoking lectures from the TED lecture series – a global conference series give voice to inspired minds. Lectures can be searched by topic, and include a number of topics in global issues, science and health. Accessed at www.ted.com

UNICEF Statistical Tables
Data on the state of the world's women and children, published by UNICEF. Browse information on maternal and child health indicators, compare by region or country, and generate tables exportable to Excel. Found at www.unicef.org/statistics

WorldMapper
An interactive display of the world's nations, resized based on the topics of interest, including social, economic, health and other indicators. Accessed at http://www.worldmapper.org/

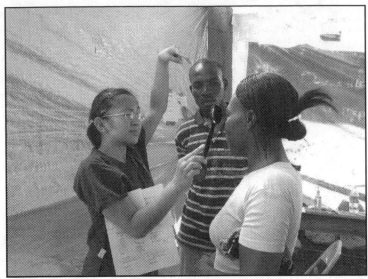

Irene Pulido, Western University of Health Sciences College of Optometry second year student, performing confrontation visual field test in Bezin, Haiti. (Photo credit: Connie Tsai)

Global Health Bibliography

The Global Health Education Consortium has produced a global health bibliography, available at http://globalhealtheducation.org/aboutus/Pages/ProjectsServices.aspx#1, last updated in January 2008. There are 830+ references in more than 25 different categories. A number of good basic textbooks are currently available including: Understanding Global Health edited by William Markle, Melanie Fisher and Ray Smego and International Public Health, 2nd edition edited by Michael Merson, Robert Black and Anne Mills.

Global Health Websites

The Global Health Education Consortium has produced a recent update in July 2007 of
the annotated global health-related websites, accessible at
http://globalhealtheducation.org/resources/Pages/GlobalHealthOnline.aspx.
This list includes links to multinational organizations such as the World Health Organization, the Global Health Council; national bodies, such as the Centers for Disease Control and Prevention (CDC); NGO's such as Partners in Health; job field and placement opportunities; language immersion programs; and online curriculum resources, such as those mentioned above.

Film Documentaries

There are a number of wonderful documentaries and films on global health.
A short list
of global health documentaries includes:

¡Salud!. Medical Education Cooperation with Cuba, 2006.
Rx for Survival - A Global Health Challenge. WGBH Educational
Foundation and
Vulcan Productions, Inc. 2005.
A Closer Walk. Worldwide Documentaries. 2003.
Beyond Borders. Mandalay Pictures. 2003.

Language Skills Training for Faculty and Residents

Language skills are very helpful when working in international
communities. There are many programs for students and practitioners of all
levels to improve linguistic ability. A guide to courses and texts can be
found at
http://globalhealtheducation.org/resources/Pages/ForeignLanguageStudy.as
px

Field Training, Courses, and Certificate Programs in Global Health

Examples of some of the many training programs relevant to faculty and
residents interested in global health are listed below. Cost (given in US $
unless otherwise noted), duration, and timing details are as of summer, 2010
and are subject to change. Many programs offer scholarships and financial
assistance for students and practitioners who have need. A more detailed
list about degree programs, international work opportunities, and volunteer
positions is available at the GHEC website at
http://globalhealtheducation.org/resources/Pages/GlobalHealthOnline.aspx.
　　　Additionally, the Swiss non-profit Medicus Mundi has an excellent
website to search global health training opportunities at
www.globalhealthtraining.org.
　　　Opportunities may also be found through global or international
health offices at medical schools and hospitals.

Community and International Field Experiences

Clinical Medical Rotations in Ecuador
Ohio University College of Osteopathic Medicine collaborates with the
Catholic University Medical School System in Quito, Ecuador to provide
clinical rotations to visiting medical students and residents. Participants
have the opportunity for cultural and language immersion, and to work in
multiple clinical settings, including a government referral hospital, the
military hospital, and as part of a surgical brigade in a small suburban
hospital. Housing is via home stay with a family. Cost $1950 for two to
four weeks (rolling enrollment,) not including travel and food expenses.
Applications at
http://www.oucom.ohiou.edu/tdi/Clinical_Rotations/index.htm

Global Health Education Project
A series of programs hosted by Mayan Medical Aid, a US NGO, which
aims to effect change in Mayan communities in Guatemala through
collaborative sustainable health and medical projects. These programs
provide participants the opportunity for language and cultural immersion,
with didactic teaching, and to practice the information learned in a
supervised clinical setting. Participants can choose to stay from two to
eight weeks in the community of Santa Cruz La Laguna, Guatemala, and
enrollment costs between $750 and $3000 depending on length of stay
(travel, food, lodging not included). Learn at
http://mayanmedicalaid.org/global_health_ed.htm

The Gorgas Course in Clinical Tropical Medicine
Hosted by the Gorgas Memorial Institute and University of Alabama –
Birmingham, this intensive 9 week course includes lectures, case
conferences, field trips, a diagnostic laboratory and daily bedside teaching
on a 36-bed tropical medicine unit. The course is taught in English, and
based in Lima, Peru, from January to March. $6,395. More information at
http://info.dom.uab.edu/gorgas/index.html

The HELP (Health Emergencies in Large Populations) Course
An intensive course in humanitarian assistance, public health principles and
disaster epidemiology hosted by the Johns Hopkins Bloomberg School of
Public Health. The course takes place in Baltimore, MD for 3 weeks each
July, and costs $1,900 for non-academic credit application. Applications
available at http://www.jhsph.edu/refugee/education_training/help.

STEER – South Texas Environmental Education and Research
The University of Texas San Antonio School of Medicine holds this four
week course primarily for medical students, but accepts residents, PAs,
fellows, and practicing physicians as well. The curriculum aims to integrate
concepts of public health into traditional medical education by an
immersion experience in the culture, language and social environment of
the South Texas-Mexico border. Taught by a diverse group of

interdisciplinary educators. Rolling admissions for four week electives throughout the year, housing fee in 2010 is $600 plus travel, food and other course expenses. Applications and information available at http://steer.uthscsa.edu/

Tropical Disease Research Program in Ecuador
Ohio University College of Osteopathic Medicine holds this workshop, geared toward undergraduate and medical students in Ecuador during June and July. Participants learn basic principles of tropical disease research, in the context of ongoing research on Chagas Disease at the Tropical Disease Institute in Ecuador. In addition to lectures on research fundamentals, participants work as volunteer research assistants on projects such as community surveys or lab analysis. Length of stay can vary from two to six weeks, and cost is $2,650-$5,120, plus $150 program fee (not including airfare to Quito.) Learn more at www.oucom.ohiou.edu/dbms-grijalva

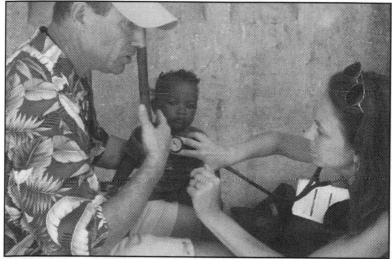

Emergency physician Dr. Wes Williams and University of Madison Wisconsin medical student Megan Shultz, discuss the pulmonary exam as they examine patient Yundy Casandra during a house call in Severet, Dominican Republic. (Photo credit: Rachel Geylin.)

Didactic and University-Based Curricula

AMSA Global Health Scholars Program
The American Medical Student Association Global Health Scholars Program is a comprehensive 7-month-long program created to inspire those medical, premedical, and public health students who are interested in pursuing internationally oriented careers in the health professions. Applications and information available at

Clinical Tropical Medicine and Parasitology Course
Conducted at the West Virginia University School of Medicine, this course
is open to physicians, residents and fellows, PAs, NPs, and public health
professionals. It focuses on the essential skills and competencies required
in clinical tropical medicine, teaches laboratory skills in a low-technology
setting, epidemiology and disease control, and traveler health. The course
is a series of four 2-week modules, and is held in Morgantown, WV during
8 weeks from June to August. Cost for all four modules is US$ 5,750 for
physicians and dentists and $4,750 for physicians working overseas for
charitable NGOs, nurses, physician assistants, and physicians in
residencies or fellowships. Learn more at www.hsc.wvu.edu/som/tropmed

Diploma in Clinical Tropical Medicine and Travelers Health
The University of Minnesota Department of Medicine hosts this 8-week,
full time, intensive training course intended for physicians and other health
care providers working in tropical medicine, travelers' health and migrant
health. The Global Health Course is offered in collaboration with the
Centers for Disease Control and Prevention as well as other local, national,
and international partners. Course prepares participants to take the
American Society of Tropical Medicine and Hygiene (ASTMH) exam for a
Certificate of Knowledge in Clinical Tropical Medicine and Travelers'
Health, and it is held in Minneapolis, Minnesota during July and August.
Enrollment fee ranges from $3,000 to $5,800 depending on degree,
employment status, and university affiliation. See
http://www.globalhealth.umn.edu/globalhlth/course.html

Diploma Course in Clinical Tropical Medicine and Travelers Health
A four month, full-time curriculum with practical instruction in tropical
medicine, including the pathophysiology, clinical features, diagnosis,
treatment, and control of diseases prevalent in the tropics. Held by Tulane
University School of Public Health and Tropical Medicine, the course is
held in New Orleans, Louisiana during 4 months from August to December.
Cost is US $10,000, plus US$1,000 for room and board. Applications and
detailed information available at
www.sph.tulane.edu/tropmed/programs/diploma.htm

Diploma in Tropical Medicine & Hygiene
This intensive, 13-week course aims to equip physicians with the
knowledge and skills needed to effectively practice medicine and promote
health in the tropics. Designed for practicing physicians, the course
encompasses four core areas: clinical tropical medicine and child health,
parasitology, vector biology, and public health. Teaching methods include
didactics, small groups, and laboratory work; and the course fulfills part of

the requirements of the American Society of Hygiene and Tropical Medicine. The course is held twice a year at the Liverpool School of Tropical Medicine, and enrollment fee in 2010 is £3,500 (~$5,400.) Learn more at http://www.liv.ac.uk/lstm/learning_teaching/post_grad/DiplTropMedHyg.htm

Diploma in Tropical Medicine & Hygiene
The London School of Hygiene & Tropical Medicine offers this three month, full time course in tropical medicine and public health, designed for physicians who intend to practice in tropical settings. The program combines practical laboratory work, a series of lectures and seminars and clinical experience, and it has been approved by the American Society of Hygiene and Tropical Medicine. The course is held in London, UK, during 3 months from January to March, and the enrollment fee in 2010 is £4,750 + £195 examination fee (~$7,600.) Find more information and applications at www.lshtm.ac.uk/prospectus/short/stmh.html

Global Health: Clinical and Community Care
University of Arizona. A multidisciplinary, case-based, problem-solving course that prepares medical students and primary care residents for health care experiences in developing countries. The course takes place in Tucson, Arizona during 3 weeks in July, and is a full-time (80 class hours), interactive course, with an optional medical/cultural weekend field trip. Free for medical students and $500 for residents and physicians, housing and textbook fees are additional. Read more at www.globalhealth.arizona.edu/IHIndex.html

Graduate Diploma Programme in Tropical Medicine and Hygiene
This full-time 6-month curriculum teaches students about tropical health problems and diseases, including epidemiology, etiology, pathogenesis, pathology, nutritional aspects, risk factors and clinical manifestations. Held by Mahidol University Bangkok School of Tropical Medicine, the course is taught in English and held in Bangkok, Thailand, during 6 months from April to September. Cost is US$4,000. See www.tm.mahidol.ac.th/en/academic/bstm/bstm_index.htm

Graduate Summer Institute of Epidemiology and Biostatistics
An array of summer courses in topics ranging from research methods and data analysis to the genetics of obesity and tobacco control, taught at the Johns Hopkins Bloomberg School of Public Health. Course durations are from one day seminars to three weeks, and non-credit tuition is $405 per credit – most courses are three to five credits. The institute is held in Baltimore, MD during 4 weeks in June/July. Data available at www.jhsph.edu/summerEpi

Principles and Practice of Tropical Medicine
The Uniformed Services University of the Health Sciences holds this course yearly, and teaches a comprehensive approach to the principles and practice of tropical medicine. The course qualifies participants to sit for the American Society of Tropical Medicine and Hygiene certifying examination in Tropical Medicine and Traveler's Health. The course is held in Bethesda, MD during 13 weeks from February to May. Cost is $5,000 for non-government affiliated individuals, and $1,500 for members of the armed services and government health professionals. Read more at http://www.usuhs.mil/pmb/TPH/index.html

Summer Course on Refugee Issues
Held by the York University Centre for Refugee Studies, the Summer Course on Refugee and Forced Migration Issues is an internationally acclaimed eight-day course for academic and field-based practitioners working in the area of forced migration. It serves as a hub for researchers, students, service providers and policy makers to share information and ideas. Program offers postgraduate training in refugee issues for practitioners involved in refugee protection or assistance. It includes panel discussions, case studies, a simulation exercise, and lectures from international experts. Held in Toronto, Canada for one week in early summer. Enrollment fee in 2010 is CAN $975 (US$922.) Course fee does not include food, travel or accommodations. Read more at www.yorku.ca/crs/summer.htm

Summer Institute in Reproductive Health and Development
Hosted by the Bill and Melinda Gates institute at Johns Hopkins Bloomberg School of Public Health, this course is aimed at mid-career professionals working in population, reproductive health and development programs in developing countries and provides training in reproductive health research and leadership skills. Held for two weeks in early summer, the 2010 enrollment fee was $2,586 (not including housing.) Learn more at http://www.jhsph.edu/gatesinstitute/education_training/workshops_training/summer_institute/index.html

Summer Institute in Tropical Medicine and Public Health
Hosted by the Johns Hopkins Bloomberg School of Public Health, this set of four two week modules provides training in tropical medicine and related public health issues. It is geared toward preparing participants to work on health problems in developing countries and with international travelers. Held in Baltimore, MD during 8 weeks from June to August (participants can take any or all of the two-week modules). Modules can be taken separately, each module enrollment fee is $1,450 (not including housing). Applications and information at http://www.jhsph.edu/tropic

214

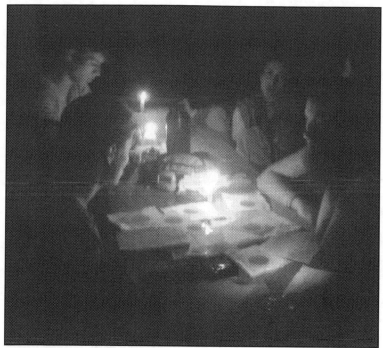

High school student volunteers with the NGO Bridges to Community review
gram stains of community water source testing by candlelight in the North
Atlantic Autonomous Region of Nicaragua. (Photo credit: Matthew Kutcher.)

Global Health Conferences

The following list details some of the larger global health conferences with
updated details as of 2010. Note that dates and websites may change.
Conferences are listed chronologically in order of yearly schedule.

The Mount Sinai Global Health Conference
Hosted by the Mount Sinai School of Medicine Global Health Center
Location: New York City
Month: February
Website: http://mssm-ghc.org

Global Health Education Consortium Conference
Sponsored by GHEC and partner institutions
Location: Rotates in North America and Central America
Month: February-April
Website: http://globalhealtheducation.org

Western Regional International Health Conference

Sponsored by the University of Washington and partner institutions in the Western US and Canada
Location: Alternates yearly from University of Washington to a partner institution
Month: April
Website: http://depts.washington.edu/deptgh/index.php

Unite for Sight International Health Conference
Sponsored by Unite for Sight
Location: Rotates in the United States
Month: April
Website: http://www.uniteforsight.org

International Conference on Global Health
Hosted by the Global Health Council
Location: Washington D.C.
Month: May-June
Website: http://www.globalhealth.org/

Doctors for Global Health General Assembly
Hosted by Doctors for Global Health
Location: Rotates nationally in the United States, next in Los Angeles
Month: July-August, every two years
Website: http://www.dghonline.org/

International AIDS Conference
Hosted by the International AIDS Society
Location: Rotates globally
Month: July-August
Website: www.iasociety.org

WONCA Rural Health Conference
Sponsored by WONCA – the World Organization of Family Doctors
Location: Rotates globally
Month: September
Website: http://www.globalfamilydoctor.com

Bay Area Global Health Summit
Hosted by University of California San Francisco Global Health Sciences Group
Location: San Francisco
Month: October
Website: http://globalhealthsciences.ucsf.edu

Canadian Conference on International Health
Hosted by the Canadian Society for International Health

Location: Ottawa, Canada
Month: October-November
Website: http://www.csih.org

American Public Health Association Annual Meeting and Exposition
Sponsored by the American Public Health Association
Location: Rotates in the United States
Month: November
Website: www.apha.org/meetings

Annual Meeting of the American Society for Tropical Medicine and Hygiene
Hosted by the American Society for Tropical Medicine and Hygiene
Location: Rotating in the United States
Month: November
Website: www.astmh.org

Consortium of Universities for Global Health (CUGH)
Hosted by CUGH, with partners GHEC and the Canadian Society for International Health
Location: rotates in Canada, next in Montreal, Quebec
Month: November
Website: http://cugh.org/meetings/annual

About the Editors

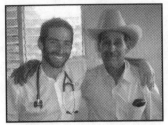

Jack Chase, MD is a family physician in San Francisco and a graduate of the University of California San Francisco Family and Community Medicine Residency at San Francisco General Hospital. During residency, he was a member of the Global Health Clinical Scholars program at UCSF. He currently works in the San Francisco Bay Area as a hospitalist and urgent care provider, and in ongoing public health projects to improve health care access in rural Nicaragua and to enhance family planning services for underserved women in San Francisco.

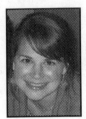

Jessica Evert, MD attended Ohio State University College of Medicine, she completed residency at University of California, San Francisco in the Department of Family and Community Medicine and participated in UCSF's Global Health Clinical Scholars Program. Dr. Evert currently serves as Medical Director Child Family Health International and is the 2010 recipient of GHEC's Christopher Krogh Award for service to underserved patients domestically and internationally.

Acknowledgments

We wish to thank, first and foremost, the many physicians, nurses, physician assistants, allied health professionals and educators who donated their time and expertise as authors and consultants on this guidebook. Their wisdom, practice, research and thought help to guide current and future global health clinicians and educators.

We would like to thank the Global Health Education Consortium, and specifically, the GHEC Executive Director, Tom Hall, for financial and institutional support of this project.

To our families, friends, teachers, colleagues and mentors, we thank you for your guidance, companionship, support and love.